Surviving
The
Death Sentence

How My Mother Survived
Pancreatic Cancer

Traysiah Spring

Dedication

This is for you
Mom

You have been a constant inspiration to me,
my whole life.

You are a powerhouse of strength and determination
and I deeply love and appreciate you, everyday.

Acknowledgements

To

Dr.'s Brian and Anna Maria Clement
and everyone at the
Hippocrates Health Institute

and

Everyone at the
Optimum Health Institute

I am grateful beyond words to you all -
for saving my mother's life.

Contents

Chapter One

The Death Sentence

The call came at 4:13am, a time when it's either a heavy breather on the other end of the line, or the news of someone dying. As I was picking up the phone, half asleep, I hoped for the obscene breather.

But it was my sister, Terri-Lee, calling with the news of our mother's diagnosis of Pancreatic Cancer. She was calling from three time zones east of me and, in her grief, had forgotten the time difference.

"The doctors give her only three months to live!" She said, trying to keep her voice steady.

Terri-Lee had always been good in a crisis, being the oldest of us five daughters. She was the one that would go into dead calm mode, when anything went wrong, and then proceed to tell everyone what to do.

"Can you come?" Her voice began to give way to a flood of sadness.

I flew out the next day, packing up my two year old son and his pile of toys and kissing my husband good-bye, as I ran out the door of our California abode.

This news came from out of the blue. I tried to piece it all together in my mind, as I gazed in a daze out at a sea of blackening clouds, spreading out below the wingspan of our 747.

My son, Jaydon, was falling asleep in the seat beside me, so I finally had a moment to myself to ponder it all, as we soared towards a foreboding future.

My mother, Samantha, used to always say, "I'm going to live to be a hundred". It was a bold statement that she would often exclaim with a glint in her eye and a cheeky smile.

But she was never one to talk about her health. Whenever you would ask her how she was feeling – "fine" – would be the only answer you would ever get out of her.

She had been in a state of exhaustion since she gave birth to five girls in three and a half years, the last birth being twins.

Then she raised them single handedly, as my father was the unfortunate combination of being a

---

10

workaholic during the week and a golfaholic on the weekends. And when we did see him, it was just the top of his head showing from behind a newspaper.

My mother's physiology never quite recovered from the many years of lack of sleep or time to herself, and over the decades she grew tired of saying she was tired, and so stopped talking about how she felt.

And she never once let on that she was going through anything out of the ordinary in these last few months.

She has been a busy and successful real estate agent for many years and as far as she let on, it was business as usual. Little did I know.

Reunion

I don't know how long it had been since all five sisters had come together from across the continent to meet again – back in our old hometown of Toronto, Canada.

When we all first arrived and saw my mother, in August of 1999, we knew that the doctors weren't exaggerating with their three month life limit.

I didn't recognize her, myself. My beautiful mother, who had once been a stunning, tall and curvaceous model, just a few years before, was skeletal thin and a definite shade of green.

She was bed ridden, emaciated and writhing in excruciating pain. Apparently Pancreatic Cancer is one of the most painful cancers to have, as the pancreas is dead in the center of all the organs and the tumor pushes hard on all of them. She said it was like someone stabbing her with a knife, again and again.

My mother refused to take any painkillers, as they made her even more nauseous. And so she just writhed in pain and moaned helplessly. Only stopping when she was forced to rush to the bathroom and violently heave the empty contents of her stomach.

At that moment, seeing her this way, I believed the Doctor's prognosis. I believed that there was no way that my beloved mother would ever come back from this state and be able to live a full life again.

My saddened heart was saying good-bye to one of my best friends and favorite people of my life. At that time, I thought that three months was generous, and I wondered if she would even make it through the night. She was definitely not going to make it to her goal of 'living to be a hundred'.

Many months before, my mother knew something was out of sorts, but she had always abhorred going to the doctor, and so avoided it as long as possible.

When she did finally hobble into the doctor's office, they checked her over and even did a full panel of blood tests, but said they couldn't find anything wrong and sent her home.

Well, as much as she detested the medical profession, she knew there was something not quite right going on in her physiology and she returned again and again for several months, but nothing was showing up in the tests and they always sent her home, saying she was fine.

Then, eight months later, after months of experiencing stabbing pains, extreme fatigue and nausea, my mother went back to her doctor and absolutely insisted that they do more tests on her.

Reticently, her doctor finally agreed to do an ultrasound and it was then that they finally found some inkling of what was causing her discomfort.

After finding this evidence of a more serious condition, the top doctors of the Toronto General Hospital stepped in to do a full battery of tests, including another ultrasound, an MRI, and not one, but two biopsies, to make sure.

Then, one of the top Pancreatic Cancer Specialists in Canada, sat my mother down and showed her the ultrasound picture of the ten centimeter in diameter (about the size of a small orange) malignant tumor sitting proudly, right on her pancreas. He informed her that there was nothing that he could do for her, as it was too large to surgically remove, and although radiation and chemotherapy may help a little, the cancer was too far advanced for these treatments to have any real effect on lengthening her life.

And then, in his best authoritative demeanor, the doctor looked straight into my mother's eyes and announced her death sentence – "Go home and put your affairs in order, you have only three months to live".

Little did we know at the time, that Pancreatic Cancer is considered to be a death sentence. Only three percent of people diagnosed with this type of cancer survive more than a year. And the three percent are usually on a morphine drip for the remainder of their excruciating existence.

Well, after the initial shock that my five sisters and I had on our arrival, we all decided not to waste another moment on moaning, ourselves. And we got to work.

All of us – Terri-Lee, Traysiah (myself), Lesley and the twins – Dawn and Dale, happened to be trained in various forms of energy healing techniques. We grew up exposed to natural healing methods, thanks to our dear mother, and now we could return the favor and put our training to good use.

We each did a different form of energy work, from Reiki to Healing Hands, where basically you allow yourself to become a healing energy receptacle and then direct the healing energy through your hands to the recipient.

Well, we all took our positions around my mother's bed, some preferred to sit, some to stand, and we proceeded to do our very best version of healing. It was powerful to have five people, who loved someone so very much, direct all of their love and healing energy towards them in silence for many hours at a time.

We would go for 2 hours, then 4, then 6. It got more and more powerful each day that we continued, and after about a week we started to see some definite changes. My mother stopped having to rush to the bathroom, and her moaning was a lot less.

By the end of the second week, her color was a little better and she could actually keep some food down. She had the strength to walk around and even started to laugh again.

We were all amazed at the power of the healing energy that seemed to be created by our "force of five". It really showed how effective energy healing could be, especially when done in a group and by people with love in their hearts for the recipient.

It was a powerful healing time for us all, as it was the first time in many years that we were all together again and we spent many hours sitting around the living room, sharing our greatest memories of our mother growing up. We had the chance to express how much we loved and appreciated all that she had done for us, and also, how much we appreciated having each other.

It was at that time, that my mother first mentioned something about a natural health clinic in Florida, called the 'Hippocrates Health Institute'. She had been researching alternative health options and had heard that this institute had been around for over fifty years and has helped thousands of people with serious health challenges, using only natural means.

It sounded great, but I really didn't think she would be strong enough to fly down. But after another week of our energy healing efforts, she had even more signs of recovery. Her color was just about back to normal and her stabbing pain had almost completely subsided.

She was still in a very weakened state, though, and I couldn't image her traveling in that condition. But she had always had a stubborn streak running though her and she started to dig in her heals, and insist on going. She wasn't quite ready to give up on her life, just yet.

The Hippocrates Health Institute was expensive – almost four thousand dollars per week, and my sisters and I had already spent so much on coming to visit my mother, some of us missing several weeks of work, and so none of us could afford to go with her to Florida, at that time. And my mother only had enough room on her credit card for herself to go down for a few weeks.

We were all deeply concerned about her going alone, but there was no stopping my mother, once she decided on doing something.

As we went to the airport with her and said our good-bye's, we all watched with heavy hearts as her frail frame walked away, and we couldn't help but wonder if it would be the last time we would ever see our beloved mother alive.

But once she arrived in the sunshine state, she was in good hands. The kind people of 'Hippocrates Health Institute' took her in and indoctrinated my mother, Samantha Young, into the wondrous world of Raw Food and Wheat Grass Juice.

Chapter Two

From Hopeless to Hope

"While there is life, there is hope."
- Stephen Hawking

Something happens when you are told that you have only three months left to live, that there is no way you can possibly survive the condition that you have.

For my mother, Samantha, who had always been a positive and tenacious thinker, something deflated inside of her. She said that it felt as if someone had punctured her life force, like a balloon, and it was draining out of her, with no help anywhere to stop it.

She was left with a deep penetrating feeling of despair and hopelessness, with nowhere to turn and nothing left to hang on to.

She had never been afraid of death, until now, when it was fast approaching like a locomotive at high speed and she was standing helplessly on the railroad tracks.

This, of course, was exacerbated by the scientific statistics, that only three percent of people have ever lived more than a year with Pancreatic Cancer. And also by the top Doctors in the country, who told her that they never expected to see her again, and that she should go home and die quietly.

Well fortunately, my mother was never one to do what she was told, and she was not about to go home and die quietly.

Although she had hardly any strength left and not one glimmer of hope, she bravely boarded a plane, all by herself, that was headed down to a place she had never been. I am still in awe of the courage and inner strength that it took for my mother to do that, in her condition.

And when she arrived in West Palm Beach, Florida, in August, 1999, it truly opened up a whole new world for her.

'Hippocrates Health Institute' is a reality unto itself. It has been around since 1956 and has helped thousands of people overcome many different serious illnesses and yet most people in the general public have never heard of it, or of the programs that it offers.

It was originally started by one of the great pioneers of natural health – Ann Wigmore – who discovered the great healing power of wheat grass juice, many decades before. And when Ann passed away, Dr.'s Brian and Anna Maria Clement took over the Institute and have faithfully carried the torch of Ann's great discoveries, ever since.

The Institute's message is, "let food be your medicine and medicine be your food". This may seem like a modern day idea, but this is a 2,000 year old quote from the ancient Greek physician, Hippocrates, the namesake of the Institute.

Hippocrates taught that wholesome, natural food could help restore physical health. Ironically, even though his original teachings were holistic, he is now remembered primarily as the father of Western Medicine.

The First Glimmer

"Once you choose hope, anything's possible."
- Christopher Reeve

When my mother, Samantha, first arrived at the Institute, Dr.'s Brian and Anna Maria Clement heard about her serious condition and they personally took her aside and told her with great certainty, "If you follow this program to the letter, for two years, you will regain your health."

Well, my mother, Samantha, was flabbergasted by this bold statement and didn't know quite what to think of it. It sounded great, but how could it possibly be true, when everyone else was saying the exact opposite.

Then they said something even bolder, "And when you go back to your Doctors, they won't believe that you're still alive and will probably say that you were misdiagnosed in the first place, even if they have the original ultrasound of your tumor in their hands."

My mother was in a state of shock and awe of what they were telling her. But it was the first ray of something other than doom, she had been given since her diagnosis, and she was grateful for even the tiniest possibility of hope.

The Clements' were especially pleased that she had not had Chemo or Radiation treatments, as that would have weakened her immune system even more, and made her recovery much more challenging, if not impossible.

Live Blood Analysis

One of the first things that they did when my mother first arrived, was a blood test called – a live blood analysis.

A 'live blood analysis' is where they take a small amount of blood and immediately put it under a microscope and observe what is actually going on in your blood at that moment.

You can see all sorts of things in your blood. You can see if there are parasites, sugar, toxins, if your immune system is working properly and many other things.

When my mother saw what her blood looked like, she was fascinated. She saw that her blood cells were all clumped together in a line. She said that they looked like groups of bubbles that were linked together in a chain.

She was told that this meant her blood cells were not flowing properly and therefore were not able to function very well.

Blood cells need to be separate and have some space to function and flow easily. So Samantha was seeing with her own eyes that her body, at the cellular level, was coagulating and breaking down in its functioning.

She was told that if she adhered to the program at the Institute, that she would see a major difference in her blood cells after a few weeks.

 My mother wasn't sure if she was going to live long enough to see the changes, but she was there to give it a serious try.

Following the Program

So what does "following the program to the letter" mean? Well, here is a basic outline -

1) Food - Eating only organic live, raw food, sprouts and green juices
2) Fasting - Doing a green juice fast for a few of days
3) Exercise - Doing light exercise everyday - lymphatic draining and stretching exercises
4) Tests - Doing live blood analysis and other tests
5) Treatments - Having massage and Far Infrared treatments
6) Colon Cleanse - Doing enemas or colonics everyday
7) Classes - Attending classes on many topics of health and nutrition – especially how to take full responsibility for your health
8) Mind/Emotions – Classes and exercises to reprogram old negative thoughts and emotions into positive and healthy ones
9) Wheat Grass Juice - And the most important and the most difficult thing of all (for my mother) was drinking wheat grass juice several times a day.

Thread of Life

"The human spirit is stronger than anything that can happen to it." - C.C. Scott

Well, even with the promise of this new program and a new glimmer of hope, my mother wasn't sure if she was going to make it through the first week.

She had started to feel better, when she was back at home in Canada, with the energy healings of "the force of five". But now that she was alone and on this new regime, she started to feel worse again.

She was told that this was to be expected, as the first part of the program usually entails deep purification as the healing process begins. And when you first start to purify you feel much worse, before you feel better. And she would have to purify in extreme measures in order to heal from such a severe illness.

But knowing this didn't help when she was, once again, experiencing extreme stabbing pain, nausea, fatigue and even emotional depression. She could hardly get out of bed the first week and could only keep down a small amount of the green vegetable juice.

She forced herself to at least go to some of the massage and colonics treatments, but otherwise, she was in bed.

She was all alone and in excruciating pain all the time. And she described to us later, that she felt as if she was really on the edge of whether she would live or die.

There were days when she definitely was ready to let go. She felt there was no point in going on, if this was the pain she had to live with.

It was as if there was only a thin thread that was holding her to life, and it could be snipped at any moment. She felt so weakened and deflated of life force that some nights when she went to bed, she really didn't expect to wake up the next morning.

When we talked to her on the phone, at that time, she sounded so frail and lost. It was very painful for my sisters and me not to be able to go and be with her at this time, and we really were very concerned that she may not make it through the week.

But somehow she did. She kept waking up, and kept living, day after day. She lived through the stabbing pain, the nausea and the fatigue. She survived the deep despair and depression.

She still doesn't know how she got through those days, but somehow, some way, she managed to hang on. It was definitely beyond her, she said. It was a divine intervention that kept her alive.

Later on, she said that she had no idea what she was capable of enduring, until she was put through this whole ordeal. It has given her a new sense of her own inner strength.

Chapter Three

Live Raw Food

"The food you eat can be either the safest and most powerful form of medicine, or the slowest form of poison." – Ann Wigmore

The second week, thankfully, my mother, Samantha started to feel a little better. She had a little more energy and was able to get out of bed for longer periods. She was even able to eat some of the raw food, but she was still feeling extremely frail and weak.

The raw food buffet was an amazing array of fresh organic vegetables, sprouts, seeds and nuts, raw soups, seed cheeses, raw dehydrated crackers, fresh guacamole and many more living raw delectables.

The buffet was actually very beautiful to behold, as my mother described it. The spread they put out at every meal, gave the feeling of being at an abundant farmer's market of 'fresh from the field' food.

My mother said that she really never felt deprived with the food, because there was such an abundance, with so much color and variety. And it was so fresh and delicious.

My mother had no idea that you could prepare so many different things and still have it considered to be raw and so good for you. It was an eye opening experience for her.

My mother had always been a beef lover from way back, and loved the 'outside cut' of roast beef with a generous side of potatoes. Any kind of potatoes would do - roasted, baked, mashed - she just loved her potatoes. So this new way of eating was an extreme departure for her, and she had a little challenge adjusting. But overall, she was surprised at how easily she started to enjoy it.

She realized that she actually did feel better after she ate this fresh food and she started to have a little more energy every day. She hadn't realized how much she was affected by the food she ate. And now she was learning to eat all over again, like a new baby. And this time she was learning to eat to 'feel good' in her body for the whole day, not just to 'taste good' in her mouth for a few minutes.

The reason why raw, living food is so good for the body is that it is still alive. It still has the life force or living enzymes pulsating through it, which means that if you were to plant it in the ground, it would still grow. So when we eat living food, this life force provides more life and energy for our body.

Whereas when we eat food that is cooked above105 degrees F., it destroys the enzymes and kills the life of the food. The energy of the food is therefore more stagnant and heavy and when we digest it, it drains energy from the body rather then provides new energy.

Cooked food also uses up our body's own store of enzymes to digest it. And our body's supply of enzymes is precious, because we are born with only a certain amount that we have to use for our whole life. And once we get low on enzymes, then we have more difficulty digesting and assimilating food.

Cooked food also has a much lower nutritional content than living food, as most of the nutrients are found in the life force of the enzymes.

So dead food takes energy from the body, while living food gives vital energy to the body. This is why it is so powerful in helping the body to heal, because it gives the body the life force and nutrients it needs to combat any imbalances that are there. The body is reminded of how it feels to be fully alive and functional again.

For my mother, it was a whole new way of thinking of food - food as fuel for the body for it's highest functioning, not just for enjoyment of the taste buds.

Our complex nervous system is like a high performance sports car. If we put junky, lifeless fuel in the gas tank of a Ferrari, for example, then it will sputter and hardly respond. What a waste of a magnificent machine that would be.

But if we put the highest quality, purest fuel in its engine, then it has the chance to perform at its peak capacity of speed, power and maneuverability.

Well, our human body, the vehicle for our spirit, has the most powerful, complex and refined nervous system on the earth. And if we fuel it properly, it can function as powerfully as a high performance sports car.

Samantha was reminded, that if we continuously fuel our refined nervous system with junky, processed, lifeless food, then our bodies will function more like a broken down jalopy.

My mother had to ask herself, then - what would she like to have for her vehicle in this life - a Ferrari or a jalopy? The choice was hers at every meal.

Samantha was re-learning to make the choice to eat the foods that made her feel more alive, and not closer to death.

And even though, she had almost no appetite at first, she was eager to try the delicious array of things from the buffet. And little by little she was able to eat more each day and keep it down.

The Hot House

It was about that time that Samantha was introduced to the Far Infrared Treatments. She was put under a Far Infrared "Hot House" Dome for an hour every day (see the back cover for a picture of Samantha under the "Hot House").

This was in 1999 and she had never heard about Far Infrared Technology before. It was very new in North America back then, but it had been used in Japan for over 30 years.

Samantha learned that the frequency of Far Infrared (FIR) wavelengths has a natural healing effect on the human body and actually accelerates the healing process. It does this in three main ways:

1) FIR detoxes our cells. The frequency of FIR resonates with the cells and causes them to release harmful toxins that have been trapped. These toxins may contribute to the triggering of disease.

2) FIR increases blood circulation. The deeply penetrating heat of FIR dilates the blood vessels, which helps to open blockages and bring more oxygen and nutrients to the whole body. This can be a big help in relief of pain, stiffness and inflammation.

3) FIR stimulates the lymphatic and immune systems, to allow the body to heal itself and maintain proper functioning.

Scientists in China and Japan have been doing research on FIR for over 30 years. In Japan it's the first treatment used in hospitals for treating many disorders, including tumors.

The Far Infrared "Hot House" Dome that is used at Hippocrates comes from Japan and has a specially arched design that maximizes the penetrating radiant heat absorbed by the body.

All Samantha knew about these treatments, at the time, was that they really helped to ease her pain and discomfort right away. She looked forward to these treatments everyday and felt so much better afterwards, and she feels strongly that they were a major factor in helping her to recover.

In fact, she loved "The Hot House" so much that when she went home, she bought one for herself and has been using it everyday, twice a day, ever since (see her website for more details – http://www.htesoqi.com/samanthayoung/).

"E's and I's"

Samantha also was given massage treatments to loosen up the toxins in her body and allow these toxins to be expelled through the digestive tract.

And then to clean out the digestive tract – she was given colonic treatments several times per week. This deeply cleans out the colon, which is where we hold many toxins. Sometimes, we have undigested food in there for years and it putrefies and creates all sorts of problems in our system.

So by cleaning out the body we allow it to function in a much more optimal way. Once again, it's just like a car – when you do an oil change on a regular basis, it keeps the engine running smoothly.

Imagine if we never did an oil change on our car. The inner workings of the engine would eventually get completely gummed up with dirt and seize up.

Well our bodies work in the same way and if we do regular cleanings for maintenance, then we'll get a lot more mileage out of our bodies.

On the days that Samantha didn't get a colonic treatment, she was instructed to give herself what they like to refer to as "E's and I's" – Enemas and Implants.

You are given a bucket and long plastic tubing and shown how to give yourself an enema (a tricky maneuver at the best of times). Then you are instructed to also do an "implant". This is where you do a smaller enema with only wheat grass juice and then try to hold it in as long as possible.

This has a powerful effect of deep inner cleansing and also helps to replenish the nutrients into the body through the colon.

This all sounds great, until you try to maneuver in a small bathroom with a large bucket, a hose and wheat grass juice. My mother had an even more difficult time of it, as she was in a weakened physical state.

She said it was like a comedy routine in the bathroom and she was glad she could lock the door. She would find herself laughing hysterically one minute, and then in extreme frustration, the next. She said the bathroom looked like a green 'Pearl Harbor' after she was done, and it took her longer to clean up afterwards, then it did to do the enema.

But in the end, it was worth the effort, as cleaning out the colon is a large part of the effectiveness of the program. And she started to feel lighter and cleaner inside her body and realized that it was giving her system a chance to heal from the inside out.

Chapter Four

Wheat Grass Juice

*"The Grass Juice Factor – a mysterious
beneficial power." – Dr. Charles Schnabel*

But the most important part of the program, was the
hardest part for Samantha. It made the "E's and I's"
seem like a walk in the park, in comparison - the
dreaded – "drinking of the wheatgrass juice".

As part of the program, she was supposed to drink
two ounces of wheat grass juice, twice a day. Two
ounces may not sound like much, but wheat grass
juice has a powerful potency all it's own.

In fact for the first while, whenever my mother was anywhere near the area where they did the wheat grass juicing, and she caught a whiff of it, she would instantly feel nauseous and have to keep walking by - quickly.

It took some time for her to actually be able to be in the vicinity of wheat grass juice, let alone be able to drink it and keep it down.

But Samantha learned that wheat grass juice is an important part of the program of healing at the Institute because of its unique curative properties.

Wheat Grass Juice Properties -

- Nutrition - One of the most nutrient dense foods available – Scientific studies show that one ounce of wheatgrass juice has the same nutrient content as twenty-three ounces of vegetables – a ratio of 1:23
- Vitamins – It contains at least 13 vitamins, including B12, C, E & A
- Minerals and Trace Elements - It has over 92 minerals and trace elements, including selenium
- Protein - It is a complete protein, containing 20 amino acids and has a higher protein density than any other food source
- Live Enzymes - It has more than 30 living enzymes
- It is also high in antioxidants and essential fatty acids

- Chlorophyll - The juice is 70% chlorophyll and the chlorophyll molecule is almost identical to hemoglobin (red blood cells) and wheat grass juice is directly absorbed by the blood and will help to rejuvenate it
- Liquid Oxygen – The juice contains liquid oxygen that is directly absorbed by the blood
- Powerful Detoxifier – detoxes the organs and blood, neutralizes toxins, protects from carcinogens
- The "Grass Juice Factor" was termed by Dr. Schnabel, an American Scientist, to describe the special beneficial powers found only in wheat grass
- Healing Accelerator – This combination of these exceptional qualities in one substance has proven to be a potent healing accelerator

Ann Wigmore, one of the great pioneers of natural health, discovered these factors about wheat grass juice, over five decades ago. Her story is fascinating.

Ann was born in Lithuania in 1909, and her grandmother was the village doctor. Ann used to watch her grandmother as she treated wounded soldiers with herbs and natural remedies during the First World War.

Ann, then moved to the United States and unfortunately, over the next several years, suffered from many different ailments, including colon cancer.

Conventional medicine was not helping her to recover from her illnesses and so she started to recall her grandmother's natural treatments and began experimenting on herself using wild weeds, herbs and greens.

Then she had an interesting experience. This is a passage from her book, 'Why Suffer - How I Overcame Illness and Pain Naturally'. (http://www.amazon.com/Why-Suffer-Overcame-Illness-Naturally/dp/0895292866)

"Seated in my bedroom, I opened my Bible to the Book of Daniel, in the Old Testament. Here I read that the dissolute King, Nebuchadnezzar, losing his mentality and his physical well-being, was instructed by a voice from heaven to go into the fields and "eat grass as did the oxen." The monarch followed this advice and in time regained his throne, his spirituality, and his physical health."

Ann took this as her own personal sign from heaven and started to concentrate on experimenting with the grasses in her area. She tried eating several different types of grass and feeding them to her animals. She noticed that both herself and her animals were thriving from the effects of one specific grass - wheat grass.

Then one day, at a local yard sale, she picked up an old cast iron meat grinder and with a few modifications, she created the very first wheatgrass juicer.

She discovered that by juicing the wheatgrass, it broke down the indigestible cellulose of the outer grass and just left the pure, nutritionally rich liquid. She then did further research with the wheat grass juice and found that it had amazing curative potency.

A few years earlier, in the 1940's, Dr. Charles Schnabel, an American scientist, was doing research on nutrition. He lead many research studies that compared the nutritional content of wheatgrass against other vegetables such as spinach, broccoli and alfalfa.

He discovered that wheat grass was the most nutrient rich of all the foods that he tested and had exceptional concentrations of vitamins, minerals, antioxidants, amino acids, essential fatty acids and enzymes.

At the time, stories about this new health food with "more vitamins than the alphabet has letters," ran in Newsweek, Business Week, and Time magazines. (http://www.rawfoodinfo.com/articles/art_wheatmeyit z.html)

In addition, his research also identified benefits from the wheat grass that could not be associated with any one of these known nutrients. The expression "grass juice factor" was termed by Dr. Schnabel, to describe the special beneficial powers found only in wheat grass.

Ann Wigmore experimented extensively on herself using wheat grass for several years, and was able to completely recover from all of her illnesses, including colon cancer.

She recounts in her book, "The change was remarkable. I came to have more energy than I ever remembered having. My weight returned to what it was in my early twenties, and my hair, which had begun to grey, returned to its normal brown color."

Then in 1956, Ann co-founded the Ann Wigmore Foundation, in Boston, MA (later to be named – the Hippocrates Health Institute). And over the next several decades, Ann helped thousands of people heal themselves using purely natural modalities.

She is now known as "the mother of living foods" and she developed a revolutionary new way of using raw enzyme-rich foods and wheat grass juice, to detoxify and heal the body, mind and spirit.

Unfortunately, at her peak of success and research, she died of smoke inhalation from a mysterious fire at her Institute in Boston on February 16, 1994.

Was the fire an accident? There are many theories about what really happened that night. Apparently Ann was a serious threat to the Western Medical Profession, as her healing discoveries were proving to be far too effective. This mystery has never been solved.

When Dr.'s Brian and Anna Maria Clement took over her Institute in Boston, they decided to move it to a warmer climate and that's when they relocated to West Palm Beach, Florida, where they have been carrying on Ann's work to this day.

The Alkaline Aha!

Another exceptional thing about wheat grass juice is that it has the same PH level as our blood. In fact wheat grass juice and live raw food are both very alkaline in their PH levels – which is a major factor of how the Hippocrates' program works so effectively, especially on cancer.

Because one of the greatest discoveries made about healing cancer is - that cancer cells cannot survive in an alkaline environment and eventually die off.

So that is one of the main reasons why wheatgrass juice and raw food are so powerful in treating cancer in a serious way, because it creates a pure alkaline environment in the body. Therefore, cancer cells, can no longer grow or survive and will eventually be killed off naturally.

Whereas if the PH level of the body is mostly acidic, then that allows all sorts of pathogens to thrive – including cancer cells, fungus, parasites, bacteria, viruses and much more.

Perhaps one of the biggest reasons why cancer and other diseases have become so rampant in society these days, is because our diet has become primarily acidic

Most of what we commonly eat now is acidic. In fact, as soon as we cook any food - it becomes more acidic. So vegetables in their raw state are alkaline, but once they are cooked, they become more acidic.

Any sort of meat product is highly acidic, including chicken and fish. Any processed foods, caffeine or sugar are also very acidic. So how does the body stand a chance in healing itself, when we pour acid into it on a regular basis?

Cancer Loves Sugar

Also, while we're mentioning sugar – cancer cells especially love to feed on sugar! This includes any form of sugar - sugar substitutes and even natural sugars from fruit. It has been scientifically verified that cancer grows much faster in an environment full of sugar.

My mother was not happy to find this out as she loved chocolate and desserts of all kinds. But fortunately, after a while, my mother found that the more she ate alkaline, non-sugary foods, the more she started to crave that kind of food. And she even got to a point of not wanting sweets or meat or anything that didn't feel really alive and healthy in her body.

Oxygenation

Another significant discovery made about cancer cells, is that they cannot survive in a highly oxygenated environment.

This has been proven in many scientific studies over the last century. In fact, in 1931, Dr. Otto Warburg won his first Nobel Prize for proving that cancer is caused by a lack of oxygen respiration in the cells.

He stated in an article titled 'The Prime Cause and Prevention of Cancer' that, "the cause of cancer is no longer a mystery, we know it occurs whenever any cell is denied 60% of its oxygen requirements."

The implication of this research is that an effective way to support the body's fight against cancer would be to get as much oxygen as you can into healthy cells. Raising the oxygen levels of normal cells would help prevent them from becoming cancerous.

Wheat grass juice has liquid oxygen in it and can easily be absorbed by the bloodstream. So it is one of the ways that can help to get needed oxygen to the cells.

These findings, that cancer cells cannot survive in a highly alkaline or oxygenated environment have been known about and verified for many years, but is a huge threat to the Western Medical Profession and to the Cancer Society, who receive billions of dollars a year for cancer treatments and research. So they have gone to great lengths to keep this under wraps.

So we will keep it our little secret... and tell as many people as we can!

Chapter Five

Self-Empowered Health

"When you make a choice, you change the future."
- Deepak Chopra

By the middle of the second week, Samantha was feeling just strong enough to start sitting in on some classes for a few minutes at a time. It was there, that she was introduced to a whole new way of looking at health.

She was shown that we are all completely responsible for our own health and only by taking full responsibility, can we be fully empowered to do something about it.

But in western society, many of us have been taught to give over the responsibility of our health to our doctors. And by doing so, we give up the ability to help ourselves. Then we are also at the mercy of what our doctors tell us – like, "you only have three months to live".

But by taking full responsibility for every choice we make in our life that may be affecting our health, then, and only then, can we have the full power to change the choices we make. And therefore change the future of our health.

My mother was resistant at first, when she heard this – to claim responsibility for creating her own ill health - but then she realized that by doing so, she could also change what she was doing and choose to create a new future for her health. A future of vital, and thriving health.

At every moment we make choices in our life. Each choice – like staying up late or going to bed early, going for a walk or watching TV, eating a bag of chips or eating organic baby carrots – each of these individual choices accumulates and comes together to form how we feel overall.

So at every moment we are unconsciously choosing either - more health, balance and bliss in the body or less health, disease and misery.

So if we decide that feeling good is more important than anything else, then all the little choices become clear.

If we have the uncompromising attitude of - "I choose everything that will make me feel more balanced, vital, alive and just plain great!" – then every choice becomes much easier.

By being aware of this, my mother realized that she had a chance to recreate a different future for herself then what she had been creating. She went from feeling like a victim of her illness, to being fully empowered to be as healthy as she chose to be.

The Amazing Healing Machine

Samantha was also reminded of the amazing healing ability of our body. One of the main functions of our body is to repair itself. It is a powerful self-healing machine.

We all know this and have experienced it. When we fell down as children and scraped our knee, our care-giver would simply clean the wound and put a bandage over it and allow the body to do its stuff.

Then, over time, we would see a scab form over the scrape and if we didn't pick at the scab, then it would eventually fall off and there would be a little pink scar where the scab used to be. The scrape would be completely healed, which was both miraculous and the most natural thing in the world, all at the same time.

We didn't have to do anything to heal it. The body's intelligence did the entire process by itself. We just needed to create the right environment for the healing to occur – by cleaning and protecting it.

That is the rule for all healing of the body. The body can heal itself from almost anything, no matter how severe, if it is given the right support and environment to do so. As long as the body hasn't been damaged beyond repair with a fatal wound.

Doctors are well aware of this rule and use it all the time. For a broken leg, they reset the bone in the correct position and then immobilize the bone with a cast. They are setting up the proper conditions for the body to heal itself.

Then they send the patient home and allow the healing process to take place. They have even noticed that when a broken bone heals, it is often stronger than it was, before the break. That is how powerful the body's healing ability is.

Doctors use this healing rule for all surgeries, as well. They know the body will repair itself after they go in and cut open areas of the body. If the body didn't have this capacity to heal itself, then the surgery would kill the patient.

But the doctors know, that if they put stitches across the incisions to hold the tissue in place, then the body will heal over these areas, and reseal itself, where it had been completely cut open and exposed.

What an amazing and miraculous thing the body's intelligence is! This intelligence is in charge of running all functions of the body. It keeps our heart beating, our lungs pumping, our blood constantly flowing, and our digestive tract and organs perpetually functioning.

It does all this, and more, all the time, without our conscious awareness. So repairing itself, is just one of the many amazing things that it is capable of.

And this self-healing capacity is run by the repair center of the body – the immune system. This is where the body regulates what needs to be done to self-repair. For a cut it is one thing, for a broken bone, it is another, for a cold or flu, it is yet another. So to have good on-going health it is vital that we have a fully functional immune system.

So why then, do western doctors completely forget this rule, of self healing of the body, and the importance of the immune system, when it comes to treating cancer?

In fact, they completely go against the body's healing process - with treatments of Chemo Therapy and Radiation - which inject highly toxic chemicals into the body that absolutely destroy the immune system.

These treatments may kill off some of the cancer cells, but they mostly destroy healthy cells, and completely compromise the immune system, making it even more difficult to recover from the cancer. The body's attention then goes to trying to get rid of the toxins, rather than to heal the cancer.

These methods are so against anything that the body has taught us for thousands of years. In fact, there are many studies that have come out in recent years that have shown that these treatments are responsible for more deaths than the cancer itself.

But giving these treatments has become such big business in North America, that many doctors are actually not allowed to offer alternatives or they can get in serious trouble.

Western Medical Treatments have become 'big business' now, but only as long as there is a demand for it.

As more and more people realize how toxic this is for their bodies, and they refuse to go along with it, and see that they don't have to poison their bodies with this "cure that is worse than the disease". Then more people will choose a healthier, more natural route, that is in tune with their body's powerful self-healing ability. And then this 'big business' will eventually be forced to go the way of the dinosaur. I hope this is sooner than later.

In future years, when we look back on this time of using these toxic treatments for cancer, it may be compared with the use of leaches and bloodletting treatments in the dark ages. It will most probably seem senseless and barbaric.

There is a great quote by Ann Wigmore –
"In this fast paced world, it is too frequently the case that people accept what society and the authorities, whom nobody ever seems to question, believe regarding how to live their lives. And yet, the happiest people I know have been those who have accepted the primary responsibility for their own spiritual and physical well-being - those who have inner strength, courage, determination, common sense and faith in the process of creating more balanced and satisfying lives for themselves."

We all know and have experienced that our bodies are powerful self-healing machines, that are born for self-repair. The body has great intelligence that can heal itself, whether it's a cut, a cold or cancer. And by working with this innate intelligence that we all have, we have the capacity to heal from anything that may be manifesting in our body. We can do this by creating the right environment that optimally supports the healing process for the body.

At Hippocrates they understand this, and my mother was seeing for herself that it is possible to heal from anything, even a death sentence, if you know how to work with your body's powerful healing intelligence.

Chapter Six

I Just Might Live

"You must find the place inside yourself
where nothing is impossible."
- Deepak Chopra

In one of the classes, Samantha learned that it takes
21 days of focus and dedication to change a habit.
And in fact, during the third week of following the
regimen as best she could, Samantha was actually
starting to feel like herself again.

She was really starting to look forward to the raw
food meals and found them to be delicious and
satisfying. And by this time she was finally able to
drink some wheat grass juice and keep it down.

Then, about the middle of the third week, one glorious morning, she woke up and looked around and thought for the first time since her diagnosis, "I might just live!"

No one was more surprised than she was, to actually be feeling like she was on the road to getting better, rather than falling down a slippery slope into disease and death.

This feeling was still fresh and new and she didn't want to jinx it, so she didn't talk about it and just nonchalantly continued doing the program of Hippocrates.

She started to have the strength to do everything on the regime. And the more she did the program 100%, the better she felt.

She even had enough energy to attend some of the exercise classes that they offered at the Institute, as well as start swimming in some of the several pools. (They have a salt pool, a cold pool, a warm swimming pool, a hot tub and a far infrared sauna.)

She also started going for long walks in their beautiful extensive grounds of over 40 acres, that are lush with tropical flowers and an organic garden.

She couldn't believe that it had been less than three weeks that she had been there and she felt so transformed from the inside out. It was amazing.

As she started to feel better and better, she was really appreciating what the Hippocrates Health Institute had to offer. She was fully realizing how simple, yet powerful the program was there. It was truly a Shangri-la for healing and she felt so fortunate to have discovered it and been able to go there – just in time.

The Clements

She was so grateful, as well, to Dr.'s Brian and Anna Maria Clement for believing in her and for creating this wonderful healing environment.

They were so encouraging to her all along, and were always available for a hug or to answer questions. Once you go there, you are treated like part of their family. They were just amazing and were truly the reason she was still alive.

Dr. Brian Clement gave a number of the lectures at the Institute while my mother was there, and she loved it whenever he did. He was such a passionate and inspirational speaker and she became a huge fan of his.

Dr. Brian Clement is an amazing natural health pioneer in his own right. He has become a world-renowned speaker about the healing power of raw food and wheat grass juice, spreading the knowledge of what he has learned from decades of treating people at the Hippocrates Health Institute.

He has overseen tens of thousands of guests at his Institute, as they have gone through amazing transformations from every kind of illness imaginable. And it has become his mission, to share what he has learned with the world.

He has also written several books and has a wonderful new website that is a wealth of information on natural health - http://therealtruthabouthealth.com.

My mother was so delighted to have met Brian and Anna Maria and they were always kind enough to give her encouraging words when they saw her. And she felt that the first words that they said to her when she first arrived, were a key part of why she got though her darkest days.

So my mother was rather taken aback when they both admitted to her in the third week, that they had been very concerned for her when she first arrived. They saw how advanced the deadly cancer was and how weak a condition she was in, and they really prayed for her that she had the strength to get through it.

My mother asked them how they could tell her with such certainty, that she would survive at that time.

They said that it was important for her to believe that she could survive. That the mind and belief system are major factors in the healing process and can make the difference between someone pulling through or not.

So they wanted to instill this belief in her right away so that it gave her a better chance to survive.

Also, it was true – that if she stuck to this program that she would have the best chance to heal.

Samantha was once again, blown away by the Clement's and the whole program there. And she realized, even more, what a miracle it was that she was still alive.

Time Moving On

It was coming to the end of the third week and my mother was coming to the end of her finances. She was feeling so much better now, than when she first arrived – her color was more white than green, and her pain had almost subsided - but she wasn't feeling quite ready to leave the healing sanctuary just yet.

She was still in a very weakened state and had a lot more healing to do. But she could no longer afford to stay.

She knew she had to say good-bye for now, but she would be back some day. She was nervous about going home, as she didn't want to go back to her old habits and start spiraling down into ill health again. But she had to trust that she had retained enough from what she had learned, that she would be able to recreate it at home.

Brian reminded her, that in order for her to continue to heal, that she had to diligently keep up this program for a full two years, at least.

It was very daunting for my mother to think of keeping up this regime at home. But she knew that she was being given the choice of life and she couldn't refuse.

Live Blood

At this time my mother was given another live blood analysis. It was amazing for her to see with her own eyes, how her blood cells had transformed over only three weeks.

She could see that her blood cells were now mostly floating around separately. They were much lighter and freer and had much more life and vitality. It was as if her blood cells were a direct reflection of how she felt now in her body.

She could see that she really had changed from the inside out.

Review

As Samantha was preparing to leave, she was reviewing all that she had learned in such a short time. This is a summary of what she learned at the Hippocrates Health Institute.

1) Raw Food and Sprouts – Filled with life force/enzymes, highly nutritious, alkaline
2) Wheat Grass Juice - Highly nutritious, potent healing benefits, alkaline
3) Alkaline Environment – Keep the PH levels of the body alkaline to kill cancer cells with raw food, sprouts and wheat grass juice. No acidic food – meat, coffee, sugar and processed foods
4) Oxygen Environment – Cancer cells cannot survive in a highly oxygenated environment and wheat grass juice has liquid oxygen that can easily be absorbed by the bloodstream
5) No Sugar – Sugar in any form feeds cancer cells
6) Detoxing – Regular massages and colonics/enemas keep the body clean
7) Far Infrared Treatments – accelerates the healing process and relieves pain
8) Exercise – Regular movement of the body keeps the energy flowing
9) Responsibility - Take full responsibility for your health – every little choice affects your health
10) Healing Power of the Body – work with the body's healing ability, not against it
11) Attitude – I can heal from anything

Continuing to Heal

On the last couple of days of her being there, she was hearing about another Natural Health Institute in San Diego, California that was similar to Hippocrates but was less expensive – the 'Optimum Health Institute'.

At the time, it was less than a thousand dollars per week and they had a scholarship program, as well, for those with life threatening illnesses.

It didn't have as nice a facility or grounds as Hippocrates. Nor did it have any extra treatments like Far Infrared, live blood analysis or full blood tests. It wasn't as personal or intimate as Hippocrates and most importantly, it didn't have Brian or Anna Maria Clement. But it had the same basic program of raw food and wheat grass juice.

Although my mother was very attached to the Hippocrates Health Institute, she knew she needed more help with healing, so she decided to give it a try.

She had to go home for a while, first, to put some things in order, but then she planned to continue her healing adventure at the other Institute in San Diego.

Saying Farewell

Samantha had one last delicious raw meal, one last Far Infrared Treatment and one last shot of wheat grass juice, then it was time to say good-bye.

She gave Brian and Anna Maria, each a big grateful hug and with a few tears, thanked them for saving her life. Then she got into a taxi and waved good-bye to one of the most amazing places she had ever been.

When my mother first arrived at Hippocrates, she really didn't believe that it was possible for her to survive, let alone, feel good and happy again.

And as she drove away, it became clear to her, that anything was truly possible. And that this was not the end, but just the beginning of her journey into healing.

Chapter Seven

Home Maintenance

"Every time you are tempted to react in the same old
way, ask if you want to be a prisoner of the past
or a pioneer of the future."
– Deepak Chopra

Arriving back home was bitter sweet for Samantha.
She was glad to be back in her lovely little house and
in familiar surroundings, but she knew she had to
make some serious changes immediately to her daily
lifestyle, before old habits started to seep in.

She immediately cleaned out her cupboards of any
processed or sugary foods - which was everything.
Then she went to an organic grocery store and bought
only fresh organic produce, sprouts and nuts and
seeds.

She had bought several raw food recipe books at the Institute and she went through the books and started to find easy to make recipes that would be satisfying for her taste buds.

She had also bought a wheat grass juicer at the Institute and found a local wheat grass grower who would deliver flats of wheat grass to her house. So she continued drinking wheat grass right away.

She also bought several other kitchen appliances that were especially good for preparing raw food – like a Vitamix blender, a dehydrator to make crackers and snacks, and a food processor for easy preparation of other recipes.

Then – her favorite thing - she researched and found where she could buy a "Hot House" Far Infrared dome, that she had become so very fond of at the Hippocrates Institute.

She decided that she wanted to not only live, but to thrive and feel great everyday. And this took a clear decision, to eat only things that supported that way of feeling.

Occasionally, she was tempted by her old habitual foods that she was used to eating her whole life – like roast beef and chocolate. But she found that even if she did allow herself to have a bite of these old favorites, that they didn't taste as good as she remembered and she felt so heavy and dull afterwards, that she started to lose interest in them.

Samantha realized that health is a decision every day, every meal, to feel in tune with your body and alive and vital or to feel dull and tired and more vulnerable to illness.

It is not up to our doctors, it is up to us. Only each one of us decides what we put in our mouths every day.

After a few weeks of integrating into this new lifestyle, Samantha was feeling fairly confident about her ability to live like this in her own life. She was really learning what worked and what didn't work for her.

But she was still feeling very weak and in need of some more deep healing.

Pancreatic Death

It was about this time, that my mother found out about two other people that had been diagnosed with Pancreatic Cancer, at the same time as she was. And they were both given the same amount of time to live as my mother - only three months.

One was a lawyer, that was only 40 years old, and he worked in the same office as my sister, Dale. He was given the three month death sentence by his doctor and then immediately packed up his desk and quit his job.

He decided to try a new experimental drug that had just come out for Pancreatic Cancer. And then, tragically, he died very quickly - within only a few weeks.

Then the other, was the father of a friend of my sister Lesley. He was told that surgery would be a good treatment for his tumor. So he went into the hospital for the operation and unfortunately never came out. He also died even sooner than his prognosis.

This made my mother realize even more, the seriousness of her illness and she thought it was time to go back into the supportive healing environment of a Health Institute. She was ready to learn more about what she needed to do, to be proactive in her own recovery.

So once again, Samantha boarded another plane to go on another adventure into healing – this time she was headed down to San Diego, California.

Chapter Eight

The Optimum Health Institute

*"You must be the change
you want to see in the world."
– Mahatma Gandhi*

The 'Optimum Health Institute' in San Diego,
California (there is also one in Austin, Texas) was
originally started as a subsidiary of 'Hippocrates
Health Institute' in the 1970's. But there were
differences of opinion of how to run the two Institutes
and so they branched off from each other and went
their separate ways. But they are both based on Ann
Wigmore's philosophies.

They both use raw food and wheat grass juice as their
fundamental healing modality and they both have
amazing, in depth classes in health and nutrition.

Optimum Health Institute or OHI, has a simpler, more self-serve type of program, as opposed to Hippocrates, that gives much more personal attention and has more healing modalities and facilities available.

But the programs are basically the same, with regards to the philosophy and the food, and are both very effective in helping to heal a wide variety of ailments or "health opportunities", as they like to phrase it.

There is no buffet at Optimum, but you are given a plate of food and can ask for a second plate if you wish. There are also no Far Infrared Treatments available, but they have massage, colonics and the blessed "E's and I's". And they have wonderful classes on digestion, nutrition, raw food preparation, and emotional, mental and physical health in general.

Optimum or OHI is different, as well, from the Hippocrates Institute, in that it is run by a non-profit church organization - a healing ministry of the Free Sacred Trinity Church, a non-denominational, Christian based church. But the program is not religious, although it does emphasize a spiritual approach.

OHI has rarely, if ever, advertised and yet, they have been full, week after week, for over 40 years by just word of mouth.

My mother adopted easily to this new Institute. She was already familiar with the raw foods and wheat grass juice and she just had to get to know the new grounds and new routine.

She really enjoyed it there, because there were a lot more people, about 100 each week, and she was meeting people from all over the world.

However, she was missing the buffet and the Far Infrared treatments, from Hippocrates. But she was so grateful to be in a healing environment again, that she just settled in and enjoyed the experience.

She still had bouts of weakness, nausea and pain, and there were days that she just stayed in bed, but mostly she was feeling much better and most importantly – was still alive!

Joining My Mother

Because it was much less expensive than Hippocrates and it was closer to where I lived in California, I was able to go to San Diego and join my mother for a couple of weeks at Optimum. So, I left my son with my husband and headed down.

It was my first indoctrination into this wondrous wheat grass world. And even though my background was in natural health (Ayurveda) and I had been a vegetarian, off and on, for years, it still was a shock to my system.

There was a big difference between eating cooked rice and vegetables, and eating all raw salads and soups, all the time. And I had always had a severe aversion to wheat grass juice.

But I was there to support my mother and to learn about this program, so I did my best to stay on the regime.

My mother had been at OHI for a week before I had arrived and she was looking amazingly well. When I first saw her, I was in shock to see how much better she looked.

I couldn't believe how much she had transformed from only about 10 weeks before - when I didn't even think she would make it through the night. She was really looking like herself again and I was completely intrigued by how this was possible.

My mother was an old pro at this raw food regime by now and was my guide as to how to navigate through it.

She showed me how to spice the raw food to make it more appetizing and how to get through the "E's and I's" without it seeming like World War III hit the bathroom. And she even helped me to juice my first wheat grass without feeling nauseous. She had come a long way in just a few weeks.

I was doing the program as best I could, but I have to admit, at first, I was strongly resistant to the whole thing. And once the purification set in after a couple of days, I went into a state of misery. I had constant headaches, overwhelming fatigue and emotional depression.

It had been the first chance I had had to deeply rest and recuperate, after being a new mother for two years, so I guess a lot of rebalancing was taking place.

My mother assured me that this was all good, and perfectly normal, but that's hard to hear when you are in the thick of it. And I was feeling rather awkward about it, as I was supposed to be there to support my mother and not to go through my own healing.

I realized, though, that if this was what I was going through, I couldn't even imagine the discomfort my mother endured when she first started the program. I gained even more respect for her.

Even though I wasn't in the best frame of mind, at first, I have to say, that I was really enjoying the classes. The teachers were exceptional and the information in the classes was so fascinating. I felt I was learning so much in such a short period of time.

My mother was such a trouper, as well. No matter how she felt, she got up everyday and went to the meals and the classes. There was even an exercise class, first thing in the morning, that she made it to more often than I did. She went to the wheat grass room and juiced her own wheat grass and even did her "E's and I's".

I was impressed with her diligence and focus. She was determined to completely recover. She was such an inspiration to me and by the fourth day, I snapped out of my resistance and I joined her full force on the program.

After I got through my initial purification, I started to feel better than I'd felt in years. I felt so light in my body and clear in my mind. I was feeling more energy than I had felt since before becoming a mother and I was remembering what it felt like to be young again.

On the fourth day, they have you go on a green juice fast for a couple of days. So you don't even get to have raw food anymore – just juice for two days. I found this challenging at first, but after the first day I felt amazing. I had so much energy and life.

Green juice fasting is a way to allow your body to rest from digestion. A lot of energy is required to digest food. Therefore, when you are fasting, that energy can be freed up to heal and rejuvenate the body. Green juice also gives the body pure nutrients that can easily be absorbed into the bloodstream.

Wow! I had no idea that you could feel such a difference in such a short period of time. I hadn't even realized how awful I had been feeling, until I felt so much better.

My background is in Ayurveda, a 5000 year old system of natural health from India. Ayurveda says that the goal of health is not just the absence of disease, but the attainment of 'Perfect Health' – the experience of complete balance and bliss in the body, mind and spirit. Well, through this program, I felt closer to that goal than I had in years.

My mother was looking better and better all the time, as well. She had truly stumbled onto an effective program for bringing back vitality to everyone, no matter what their original condition of health.

<u>Rejuvelac</u>

Another aspect of the program that I really responded to, was the freshly prepared Rejuvelac. Rejuvelac is a drink that is made from fermented sprouts that becomes a powerful probiotic. As part of the program, you drink several cups of Rejuvelac everyday and I found that my whole digestive tract felt better and calmer.

When you put healthy flora into your digestive tract, then it can balance any unhealthy microbes that may be taking over in your colon. This is a big part of overall health, because when the digestive system is working properly, the whole body functions better.

This was one thing that developed at the Optimum Institute and wasn't a part of the Hippocrates program. It became one of my favorite things about OHI.

105 - Still Alive

The second week I was really starting to enjoy their food as well. They have wonderful 100% live raw vegan meals of mock spaghetti and meatballs, tacos, sushi and even pizza. All of these meals were delicious and were all prepared using dehydrators instead of ovens, that kept the temperature under 105 degrees F.

'105 - still alive' - is a catchy phrase they use to remind us, not to heat the food above this temperature, to keep the living enzymes and life force from being destroyed.

There were many classes that demonstrated how to prepare these raw meals as well. Classes on how to use a dehydrator, how to make raw sushi, crackers and sauerkraut.

They showed us how to prepare all sorts of delicious raw recipes and it was all hands on, so you really had a chance to get a feel for doing it yourself.

Then at the end of the week, all the food that was prepared by the guests, was set out in a lovely buffet for the other guests to sample. It was a fun experience for everyone involved.

After taking these classes, my mother and I had a much more practical idea of how to recreate this lifestyle at home. And it gave us both a lot more confidence that we could do it.

Chapter Nine

Overview of Classes

*"Let food be thy medicine and
medicine be thy food." - Hippocrates*

There are three weeks worth of classes at OHI that are
packed with information and the guests are
encouraged to go through the program for three
consecutive weeks, in order to take all the classes,
and to give their body a chance to really purify and
heal in a deep way.

We learned so much in such a short period of time in
these classes, and this is a simple overview –

For optimal health and feeling great - they
recommend a simple diet for everyday life, consisting
mostly of fresh organic produce, sprouts, nuts, seeds
and whole grains.

I was happy when they suggested for most people, to have a diet that wasn't 100% raw, but to have 80% raw and 20% cooked food. This sounded a lot more practical and easy to maintain as a day-to-day lifestyle.

As for the cooked food – they suggest that it should be freshly prepared (not left overs) and simple – like steamed brown rice, quinoa, beans, lentils and chickpeas.

They also emphasize proper food combining, for optimal digestion and assimilation of food. For more information on food combining – see the last chapter – 'More Information'.

Then they went into a lot of details of what is unhealthy for the body to eat.

Processed Unfoods

I found that the foods that are considered to be unhealthy, mostly boiled down to this – any food that is processed from its original, natural state is not really food, but 'unfood'.

Processed food becomes a foreign agent to the body and can't be properly assimilated and tends to create all sorts of negative reactions and inflammation in our system.

For example – anything that comes in a box, bag, bottle or can, is most likely processed or refined from its original state. And when you eat it, may cause – fatigue, head aches, unclear mind, irritability, bloating, low energy, blood sugar spike and then drop and many other reactions.

These are all signs that your body is not happy with what you are feeding it. But most of us have been eating processed food for so long, that we have become accustomed to these reactions and we think it is a normal way of feeling after eating.

What if these reactions are not normal and we can actually feel clear, light and full of energy after eating? What a concept!

Our body is a living organism and it recognizes and is designed to digest and assimilate other living organisms. So when we eat foods that are not a living organism, then the body doesn't really know what to do with it.

But when we eat foods that are closest to their original living form, when they are picked from the fields, then our body does knows what to do with it. It can absorb the nutrients properly from these foods and easily dispose of the rest.

But with processed food, the body has to filter all the foreign, unrecognizable chemicals and sugars through the liver and other organs.

This is often why we feel tired after eating, because it takes the body extra work to process it. And these foreign chemicals in the body, also cause inflammation of the tissues, which is the precursor of all disease.

Unprocessed Shopping

So what does eating unprocessed food mean? Well this means that shopping for groceries is a lot easier – you can skip all the aisles in the grocery store that have the boxes, bags and cans, (which is most of the middle aisles) and go straight to the produce section. Which is a feast for the eyes and nose in its selection of fresh, colorful, living vegetables and fruits.

The bulk foods section also, has a healthy selection of organic raw nuts, seeds, rice, quinoa, beans, lentils, chickpeas and other natural foods in their unrefined forms.

A consolation for this way of shopping, is that it's generally cheaper to buy foods in their raw state. Processed foods in boxes and bottles, tend to cost more, as you're paying for all the work that goes into producing them.

Simplicity is the key. Eating simple, organic, clean, green, unrefined foods that are not complicated by processing, chemicals and sugars. This is what your body really craves and needs to function optimally.

Also, preparing the cooked meals fresh every time, and not having left overs or pre-prepared meals from days before.

I like to think of it as "clean, green eating" – a simple clean diet of green, unprocessed, living food that your body loves and thrives on. And makes you feel great!

And there is such a vast rainbow of variety of vegetables, fruits, nuts, seeds, beans, whole grains and infinite ways to prepare them, that you don't ever have to feel deprived with this way of eating, but can feel deliciously satisfied and vitally alive.

It is just a reorientation of what you think of as food. And after a while you don't even notice the aisles in the grocery store that you no longer go down.

Actually, after some time of eating cleaner and simpler, the boxes and cans down these aisles, no longer even seem like human food, but are more like pretty packages that decorate the shelves.

Once you start experiencing living foods, then the food in the packages, seem as lifeless and cardboard as the boxes they come in.

The List

Processed foods include – okay are you ready for this list?

This may be difficult for most people to hear, but I guess we have to ask ourselves at this point – how much do we really want to heal and feel great?

Are we willing to make changes and let go of old habits in order to experience exceptional vitality and health? Only you can decide.

Okay, well OHI just recommends having less of these things in our diet and then over time, perhaps we will crave them less and less.

Here goes –

1) Generally – Anything that has been packaged – boxed, bagged, bottled, canned, frozen and has more than one ingredient in it. Especially any chemical ingredients that you don't recognize as natural.

2) Such as – cereal, crackers, cookies, salad dressing, sauces, condiments, any canned food, deli meats, potato chips, ice cream, frozen prepared meals, boxed prepared meals and the list goes on…

3) This also includes packaged foods in the natural health section that are supposedly 'healthy' processed food, which unfortunately are just as processed as the regular processed food, no matter how much it has been fortified with vitamins

4) Wheat, bread, pasta, cakes, etc. - Anything made with refined flour is like "goo and glue" in your digestive tract

5) White Rice/Refined Grains – Refined starch that reacts like sugar in the body and the nutrients have been taken out. Instead - have brown rice and whole grains
6) Sugar – Anything with any form of sugar (including sugar substitutes) is upsetting to the blood sugar levels and the Pancreas and is toxic for the body. It also feeds cancer cells
7) Soda – Pure toxic chemicals, sugar and carbonation that dehydrates the body, strips the bones of calcium and are highly acidic
8) Prepared Drinks – Any drinks in a bottle or can that are not plain water - are processed
9) Alcohol – Highly toxic for the body – a hang-over is the body trying to expel the extreme toxins

They also mention a few more foods that are best to have less of in your diet, as well. Keep in mind that they are just suggesting to have a little less of these as part of your daily lifestyle, with the goal of feeling as vital and healthy as possible.

1) Meat – Including chicken and fish - Filled with hormones and harmful cholesterol. Decades of studies have shown that it is directly related to heart disease and cancer (See the book –'The China Study')
2) Dairy – The human body is not set up to properly digest other mammal's milk products – this includes cheese, yogurt, ice-cream. Dairy has 'casein', an animal protein, which

studies show accelerates disease, including cancer ('The China Study')

3) Coffee – Dehydrates the body, is highly acidic and the caffeine throws off the adrenal glands

Whew! Okay well we got through the lists. How did you do? For some people it's not a big deal, for other's it's catastrophic.

But even being aware of what is best for your body can start you thinking in that direction and then who knows what is possible?

A Stroll in the Garden

Let's take a break now, after those challenging lists and go for a stroll in the garden.

One of my mother and my favorite things to do at OHI was to stroll through the sizable organic garden that is planted on the grounds of OHI.

We would wander through the abundant aisles of vegetables, fruit trees and flowers and see what was in bloom and was ripe for the picking.

My mother loved to pick some flowers for her room and I loved to cut some fresh mint leaves to make mint tea.

At OHI, they use many of their own vegetables right from the garden in the preparation of meals. And during that time, they had freshly picked ripe cherry tomatoes that popped in your mouth with an explosion of flavor.

It was fun, as well, to wander by the giant green house where they grow their own trays of wheat grass. We would peak in and see row upon row of trays, in a vast sea of growing greenery.

OHI has one of the largest production facilities for growing wheat grass in North America. They go through a lot of wheat grass, with over 100 guests every week.

Chapter Ten

Cancer

"You gain strength, courage and confidence, by every experience in which you really stop to look fear in the face." - Eleanor Roosevelt

Now, it's time to tackle an even more intense subject. In the OHI classes they covered a lot of information related to cancer. This is a taste of what we learned, as well as, other things that my mother and I have discovered over the years.

So what exactly is cancer? How is it created in the first place? Well, cancer is created from perfectly normal functioning cells - that have turned bad.

Healthy cells that have become mutated somehow into cells that attack and destroy the body, rather than help support the body to run smoothly.

Why do these cells turn bad? Scientists are still researching all the possibilities. But many studies have shown, as we have mentioned earlier, that it may start by the cells being deprived of enough oxygen to function normally, and so the cells begin to mutate.

What causes this lack of oxygen in the cells? Well, it has been shown to be a build up of too many toxins and carcinogens in the body, which block and damage the cells' ability to take in and process oxygen.

Some of these toxins and carcinogens are –

1) Toxins from our environment – air, water, food, skin products
2) Genetically modified (GMO) or mutated foods
3) Animal protein in meat and dairy
4) Negative thoughts and emotions

Environmental Toxins

Environmental toxins are everywhere, all the time, in this industrial age. They are mostly from man made chemicals that are in - the air, water, food and products for our body.

Can we avoid these toxins? Not all of them, but we can make the best choices for the things we directly put into or onto our bodies – like food, drink and even skin care products and cosmetics.

Anything that we put on or in our body has an affect, even the skin care or cosmetic products that we use. Anything that we put on our skin gets absorbed into the bloodstream. The doctors know about this, as they prescribe medicated creams, in which the medication is absorbed through the skin.

So, a good rule of thumb is to think of anything that goes onto our skin, as something that we would eat. And as we become more aware of the ingredients of the skin creams, toothpaste and cosmetics that we use, then we can make more natural choices.

As for what we drink. Our bodies are made up of 100 trillion cells and each cell is mostly made of water. In order for our cells to function in their most vital way, they need to stay hydrated. So our body craves lots of fresh clean water. It is an important part of good health. At OHI it is a big part of the program to carry a water bottle with you at all times and to be drinking water all day long.

Unfortunately, when we drink anything with sugar, caffeine or chemicals in it, then we are actually dehydrating our cells and giving our body more work to do, as it will need to purify these foreign agents out of the body. So what our body really wants and needs is simply - clean fresh, filtered or bottled water.

As for food, we can choose organic. Organic food is simply produce that has not been sprayed with toxic chemicals. The irony is, that a hundred years ago everything was organic, because they hadn't discovered the toxic chemicals that are now used to spray most of our food crops.

But now they spray most of the crops with extremely toxic pesticides, herbicides and fungicides that are highly poisonous, and then they put this food in the grocery stores and say they are safe to eat.

Organic food is just food that is in its original natural state and hasn't been sprayed with these toxic chemicals. They also come from organic seeds that have never been sprayed.

And ironically, now that most of our food supply has been poisoned by these toxic sprays, there is a premium cost for organic food – that has not been poisoned.

Have you ever noticed that the rise of cancer statistics correlates perfectly with the use of insecticides on our food crops, that started in the 1950's.

I still don't understand how the farmers and scientists have not put two and two together, to realize that if the poisonous sprays are toxic to the bugs on the plants, then they will probably be toxic for the humans that eat them, as well.

Mutations

One of the most disturbing causes for cancer is the mutated organisms that we take into our bodies from unsuspecting sources. Many of our foods now are genetically engineered. They are called 'genetically modified organisms' (GMO) or in other words – they are foods that have been mutated from their natural state.

The scientists have taken the genes from one species and spliced them together with the genes of other species and created a whole new species. For example they take genes from a fish and put it together with the genes of a tomato plant and voila! They have created a tomato plant that will be more resilient when growing.

This is amazing that they can do this now, and their intention is to improve our lives, but the scientists unfortunately have not taken into consideration that these mutations may possibly affect the cells of the people who eat them.

These mutated food products go into our bodies and have been shown to induce mutation of our own cells. Statistics have shown that the sudden spike in cancer cases in recent years, directly correlates with the increase of use of GMO's in our food supply.

The most common GMO foods are – tomatoes, corn and soy, among many others. And any products made from these foods, like - tomato sauce, high fructose corn syrup, tofu and soy milk. Unless they are certified organic, they are most likely GMO.

Another thing that has been coming to the fore in recent years, is the affect of using microwave ovens. The term "nuke the food" is accurate, in that electromagnetic radiation is used to heat the food. This radiation changes or mutates the molecular structure of the food as it is heated. When we digest these mutated molecules, then they have a direct affect on our cells.

It can be overwhelming to think of all the possible toxins and mutations in our environment, so we just have to see for ourselves what works for us. Everyone is different and we each have to figure out what feels good for us.

Only we can be the true researchers of our own health. And it comes from trial and error of experiencing how we feel when we try different things. Then we can clearly choose what is right for our own vital and thriving health.

Animal Protein

This is a surprise to most people, I know it was to me, when I heard that eating meat products and even dairy, were directly linked to increasing the risk of cancer.

I knew that meat wasn't good for your heart, but cancer?

Well, this fact is painstakingly documented in the largest comprehensive study of human nutrition ever conducted – 'The China Study'. (http://www.thechinastudy.com)

This study was conducted over 20 years, beginning in 1983 and was done on 6,500 adults in 65 different counties in China. It was conducted as a partnership between Cornell University, Oxford University, and the Chinese Academy of Preventative Medicine.

It was overseen by Dr. T. Colin Campbell, who wrote the book on the study and recounts, "When we were done, we had more than 8,000 statistically significant associations between lifestyle, diet, and disease variables."

The results are irrefutable and simple - eat a plant-based diet to have good health. Dr. Campbell says, "People who ate the most animal-based foods got the most chronic disease. People who ate the most plant-based foods were the healthiest."

Animal-based food, surprisingly includes dairy. The research shows that the main protein found in cow's milk - called 'casein' - directly causes the growth of cancer cells.

Dr. Campbell grew up on a dairy farm, so he used to enjoy drinking a lot of milk. But not anymore. In multiple, peer-reviewed animal studies, the researchers discovered that they could actually turn the growth of cancer cells on and off by raising and lowering doses of 'casein'.

Another interesting finding in the study, is that the quality of nutrition in the food you eat, affects the growth of cancer. In other words if you have a nutrient rich diet of fresh produce, then the body can better fight off the effects of toxins and carcinogens in the body. And these toxins, then, don't have near as negative an influence. So this is another reason why a fresh plant-based diet is effective in fighting cancer.

Dr. Campbell stated, "The results of these, and many other studies, showed nutrition to be far more important in controlling cancer promotion than the dose of the initiating carcinogen."

Then he goes on to say, "There are virtually no nutrients in animal-based foods that are not better provided by plants."

This is even true for protein – yes, protein! There is a surprisingly large amount of protein in dark green leafy vegetables, beans, nuts and seeds. And of course - wheat grass juice.

The New York Times has recognized 'The China Study' as the "Grand Prix of epidemiology" and the "most comprehensive large study ever undertaken of the relationship between diet and the risk of developing disease."

I first heard about this study in a wonderful ground breaking film - 'Forks Over Knives' - (http://www.forksoverknives.com). Which was a life changing experience for me to watch and I recommend it highly.

My mother and I both, were powerfully moved by these findings and my mother has adopted a 100% vegetarian lifestyle, ever since. She believes that this is a big reason why she is still around.

Chapter Eleven

Mental and Emotional Health

*"Happiness is when - what you think, what you say
and what you do - are in harmony."*
– Mahatma Gandhi

Another element that has a powerful effect on cancer
risk and on health, in general, is the way we feel and
think.

If your mind and emotions are not happy, then your
body is probably just an expression of that. In order to
have complete healing, you have to look at the
underlying mental and emotional influences that may
be creating the physical manifestation.

This was the most challenging area for both my
mother and myself to truly investigate.

We all have traumas and challenges in our lives. To face these and acknowledge how they affect us, can be very painful.

I knew my mother had been upset about how my father had treated her for over twenty years. She didn't show it on the surface, but she held onto these hurt feelings deep inside. She was very resentful for years of neglect, constant put downs and general lack of support. I can't blame her for feeling these things, I was there and I saw that this was true. But by holding on to these feelings, they were literally eating away at her from the inside out.

I had my own negative thoughts/emotions that I had hidden inside of myself and I found it very difficult to dig around and bring them out to be healed.

They talked about these thoughts and feelings at OHI, as mental and emotional toxins.

Mental and Emotional Toxins

"I don't think of all the misery, but of the beauty that still remains." - Anne Frank

Mental and Emotional toxins are reoccurring negative thought patterns from old traumas from the past.

Anger, guilt, shame and resentment are the most potent of these negative thoughts/emotions and when we allow these thoughts to circulate in our awareness constantly for years, they actually create physical manifestations in many different forms.

How do we change these thought patterns? Forgiveness and letting go of them is a big part of healing this – but this is easier said than done.

Just by talking, becoming aware of and venting out these old feelings, this can really help in deflating the energy behind them. My mother and I had many deep discussions at that time about my father and about other traumas that had affected each of us. It was very helpful for both of us to express it all out in the open and feel that it was okay to feel the things we felt.

But this is only the first level of healing them. We often have to go deeper to get to the root of these feelings, in order to be finally free of them.

Blame

"Whatever relationships you have attracted in your life at this moment, are precisely the ones you need. There is a hidden meaning behind all events, and this hidden meaning is serving your own evolution."
– Deepak Chopra

Another thing they talked about in class was – blame.

When we blame anything or anyone other than ourselves for anything in life – then we are giving over our power to that person or thing. We are giving them control over whether we will recover from the incident.

Again, it comes down to taking full responsibility for our life. But how can we be responsible for bad things that have happened to us?

Well, if we think of everything that happens in our life as a learning opportunity and that we came down to this earth to learn and grow as a soul, then we can see these things as coming to us for a good reason.

If everything in life was easy and happy, then would we grow and get stronger? Not near as much as if we were tested and challenged. To have a life on this earth seems to entail having traumas and dramas, no matter how much we try to avoid them.

So if everything that happens to us is for a valuable reason and is for our growth, then it may be a waste of energy to blame the ones that bring us these circumstances. Are we not, then just "shooting the messenger"?

But, then again, it is natural to feel resentment and anger towards others that have done some offensive things to us. And when we do feel these emotions, we tend to unconsciously hold on to them, until we either get revenge for what has happened, or get an apology.

But when we can step back, way back, and look at these situations from an objective perspective, and see that we may have learned something of value from them and may have grown in ways that we would not have been able to otherwise. Then maybe we can let go of keeping track of these offenses and start to free ourselves of the heavy weight of the emotions that we carry.

It's not that we are saying that it was okay to do what they did. Not at all. But for our own health we have to let go of the toxic emotions that we have been hanging on to.

When we realize that we are not actually getting back at the other person at all, by hanging on, but instead, we are only harming ourselves, then this may help us to let go.

This was really brought home to my mother when my father past away. She was still upset about how he had treated her and she unconsciously wanted him to acknowledge and apologize for his behavior. But it never happened. He moved on to another realm and had completely forgotten about it and my mother was never going to get her apology.

She realized at that time that she had held on to those feelings for over twenty years after their divorce, and she kept the pain of that relationship going for all that time. And, yet my father didn't even give it a second thought.

She had jeopardized her health by holding onto those feelings and for what? It was time to free herself of them and free herself of her relationship with him.

Forgiveness

"People are often unreasonable and self-centered.
Forgive them anyway.
For you see, in the end, it is between you and God.
It was never between you and them."
– Mother Teresa

What is forgiveness? Is it letting people walk all over us and saying it's okay. No, but we can never control what others do, as much as we try. The only thing we can control – is our response to it. That is the only thing that we can fully control in our lives.

Viktor Frankl wrote a wonderful book, 'Man's Search For Meaning', in which he wrote about living through the horrors of a Nazi concentration camp in World War II. He learned that he may have been a prisoner in his body, but not in his mind. He experienced that no matter what was going on, he could respond in a way that felt good inside of him.
(http://www.amazon.com/Mans-Search-Meaning-Viktor-Frankl/dp/080701429X)

When he had long days of hard physical labor, he would put his attention on the love of his wife. He realized that he could feel the love they had no matter what was going on.

This was a powerful life lesson for him, to see that no matter what horrors were going on in his life, that he was free in his mind to be happy and feel love. It was only the brief moments that he allowed anger and hatred to penetrate his thoughts, that he became a prisoner once again.

The great theoretical physicist, Stephen Hawking, who is confined to his wheelchair and is completely paralyzed in his entire body from a motor neurone disease, has a wonderful quote –

"Although I cannot move and I have to speak through a computer - in my mind I am free."

We are indeed free in our mind, no matter what is going on in our lives. Perhaps we are each being tested in our own way, to see if we have learned this life lesson yet.

So what is forgiveness? Perhaps it is the freedom in our minds and hearts to choose to love and let go of anything going on in our lives that is not creating peace and happiness.

We can let others be free to do what they need to do, and that allows us to be free to think and feel what we want. What an amazing freedom that is. Then it doesn't matter what is going on in our lives, we can always choose to be happy.

Ho'oponopono

A simple technique that I have come across, has really helped me to let go and forgive in many circumstances. It's called Ho'oponopono and it originated in Hawaii and it is based on forgiving others, as you wish them to forgive you.

It is simple – you just think of the person or situation that you want to forgive and you repeat to yourself –

"I'm sorry, forgive me, thank-you, I love you."
"I'm sorry, forgive me, thank-you, I love you."
"I'm sorry, forgive me, thank-you, I love you."

You repeat this over and over again and it has a magical quality of making you feel much lighter and freer of what you are thinking about. Because, rather than forgiving them, you are asking for their forgiveness of yourself and sending them thanks and love, as well.

I have found miraculous results from this. Even in the most conflicting situations, when I do this technique,

I usually feel much more forgiving of the other person, afterwards. And I find that the other person, more often then not, has a much more open and receptive response to me.

Attitude of Gratitude

"Attitude is a little thing that makes
a big difference." - Winston Churchill

One of the simplest and most effective ways to change negative thinking into positive thinking at any moment – is to catch ourselves in mid-negative thought, and stop what we are thinking (at OHI they suggest saying to our self - "cancel, cancel" – to reset that thought pattern) and then to take a moment and remember something – that we are grateful for.

"I am grateful for… in my life." Allow our mind to go to as many things as we can think of, that we are grateful for in our whole life.

Then it's amazing how much better we can feel. Our heart can open up and connect with what truly brings us joy in our life.

One suggestion, is to think of, or write down, a list of things that we are grateful for, when we first wake up in the morning. Then we can think of our 'grateful list' all throughout the day.

After all, there is so much to be grateful for – just being alive is one of them! And this reminds us of the simple wonderfulness of life, and allows other more negative or worrisome thoughts to be put aside.

This 'attitude of gratitude' is a powerful tool to keep in our pocket at all times. It is a simple way to steer the mind towards what is really important to us in our lives, and allows the heart to flow and be open, no matter what is going on around us.

Louise Hay

"Every thought you think is creating your future!"
– Louise Hay

Another effective tool for working with our thoughts and emotions is a wonderful book by Louise Hay, called - "You Can Heal Your Life".
(http://www.louisehay.com)

Louise is another exceptional leader in natural healing and she wrote this book after helping thousands of people to heal their lives, over many years.

Louise discovered that there were common underlying mental/emotional components to each type of physical ailment and she documented these correlations. This book is a wonderful compilation of her findings.

In her book – she has a chart that you can look up many different physical ailments and see what the underlying mental/emotional thought pattern is, that is causing it. Then she offers powerful "new thought patterns" or affirmations that you can say to yourself to help create a new way of thinking.

I found this book fascinating and my mother and I looked up several things related to my mother's condition.

When we looked up - 'Pancreas' - Louise has written, "The pancreas represents the sweetness of life." Ailments of the pancreas represent – "Rejection, anger and frustration, because life seems to have lost its sweetness."

This really touched my mother and she felt it really hit home with how she has been feeling for many years.

The affirmation is - "I love and approve of myself and I alone create sweetness and joy in my life."

Then we looked up cancer. It was very intense and powerful. It says that cancer represents – "Deep hurt, longstanding resentment. Deep secret or grief eating away at the self. Carrying hatred." The overall feeling is - "What's the use?"

My mother also related to this very strongly.

The affirmation for cancer is – "I lovingly forgive and release all of the past. I choose to fill my world with joy. I love and approve of myself."

My mother adopted these new thought patterns and repeated them to herself, everyday in front of a mirror. She said that they did make her more aware of her old thoughts and then she could catch these old thoughts and retrain herself to have happier ones.

In my whole life, my mother was never one to express her emotions or even allow herself to feel them. This was such a huge step for her to acknowledge some of these things she was going through. I was really proud of her that she was ready to open up and heal herself in this way.

Visualization

Another powerful technique is using visualization to help in the healing process. This is where you close your eyes and imagine in your mind, different scenarios that can enhance the effect of healing.

There are many different visualizations and self-hypnosis imagery techniques that you can use. I have been trained in Hypnotherapy and these are a few examples that I have come across.

One example of a visualization is - picturing your 'health opportunity' or illness, dissolving away and having white or green healing light coming in to heal it.

Then imagine yourself, when you are truly healthy again and remember what that feels like. Then step into that image and feeling of health, right now.

You can also have an open discussion with your 'health opportunity' and ask it what it requires to heal and then listen carefully to the response. You can ask it many things and find out what you need to do, to facilitate its healing, as well as, what caused it in the first place.

Another way, is to visualize an ideal healing sanctuary inside of yourself and then to remember this place - what it looks and feels like. Then you can access this place anytime you want, when you close your eyes.

These are just some quick examples of visualizations. There are so many possibilities with this modality.

You may want to find a certified Hypnotherapist in your area that can lead you through some powerful visualizations and work with your subconscious mind to help you to heal.

Hypnotherapy has been shown to be a powerful accelerator in the healing process and is used in many healing clinics across the country, now.

An excellent source of information on Hypnotherapy is the Hypnosis Motivation Institute. It has a wealth of videos, CD's and a list of Hypnotherapists around the world - https://www.hypnosis.edu

EFT

There are so many techniques to help heal the mind and emotions. But I will mention one more that I have come across in recent years – The Emotional Freedom Technique (EFT).

EFT is a form of emotional acupressure, based on the same energy meridians used in traditional acupuncture, but without needles.

Instead, simple tapping with the fingertips is used to input energy onto specific meridians on the head and chest while you think about your specific emotional issue or problem.

This combination of tapping the energy meridians and feeling the blocked emotions, works to clear the "short-circuit" from your body's bio-energy system, and restores balance to your mind and body.

EFT works deeply and efficiently to help "clear out" long embedded emotional issues that may be sabotaging your life.

There are many different websites to visit for more information on EFT. Here are a couple -
http://eft.mercola.com/
http://www.rogercallahan.com/index2.php

Chapter Twelve

The Spirit

*"In the midst of movement and chaos,
keep stillness inside of you."*
- Deepak Chopra

At OHI there are many classes that talk about the
more spiritual aspect of life. They are not preaching
any specific approach to spirituality, but instead allow
open discussions on what this means to each
individual and they encourage everyone to find their
own connection to a higher source.

They emphasize that by learning to accept and love
yourself, you will gain a sense of freedom to live your
life fully and achieve optimum health.

They say, "When you awaken the spirit within you, you can better cope with pain, disappointment, and loss. In the safe and sacred environment of OHI, people from all religious traditions are able to nourish their spirit through reflection, prayer and celebration."

They encourage you to awaken your spirit by asking yourself -

- What inspires me?
- What gives me hope?
- What gives me joy?
- What touches my heart?
- What heals my heart?

Taking time to identify what is important to you is a powerful way to bring about inner and outer transformation.

This spiritual emphasis of their program is also reflected in their – five P's to cultivate healing -

- Purpose - to achieve a natural balance and reconnection to the Divine
- Positive - mental attitude that supports the healing process
- Persistence - in following the holistic disciplines of the OHI program
- Patience - with yourself as you allow your body, mind, and spirit to heal
- Prayer - to a higher source who will share the load with you.

I have found that the atmosphere at the Institute really does have a divine feeling level to it and this encourages an overall feeling of caring and nurturing for each other. This is a big part of what creates the healing environment there.

Hugs

"Hugs can do a great amount of good."
– Princess Diana

Part of what creates the nurturing environment there, is that before each meal, all the guests are invited to join in a big circle and hold hands and hear some inspirational words that are read by a program leader.

Then they all repeat some uplifting words together and let go of their hands and hug themselves and then each other.

At first, I was a little wary of this 'touchy-feely' ritual, as I am not inclined to join in on these kinds of things. But when I finally ventured to join in a few times, I was so warmed by the experience, that I started to go as often as I could.

They even have 'designated huggers' at the Institute. These are guests that volunteer to give hugs to those who look like they are in need of a little love.

It's amazing how something so simple as getting a hug when you could really use it, can make you feel so much better.

Meditation

There are several classes in meditation, relaxation and yoga stretches, as well, that are very helpful.

My mother and I, both, have had many years of experience with meditation. My mother brought our whole family to learn to meditate (Transcendental Meditation) when I was just a child. I had such a deep experience right away, that I have kept meditating ever since and now it has been over 38 years.

We both meditate every day in the morning and evening. As soon as we wake up in the morning we just sit up and close our eyes and go inside to a lovely place of silence.

It is a wonderful way to connect with something greater than yourself, before you get involved with the distractions of the day.

For myself, it has been a lifesaver in so many ways and I don't know how I would have gotten along in my life without it. It is one of the many things that I am forever grateful to my mother for – for introducing me to it.

I cannot recommend enough, giving some time to your self, everyday in complete silence and stillness.

It allows all parts of your self – mind, emotions, body and spirit - to heal and rejuvenate at a profound level.

Chapter Thirteen

Transformation

*"The measure of intelligence
is the ability to change."*
- Albert Einstein

The whole experience at the Optimum Health
Institute was eye opening for me in so many ways.
One of the things that was fascinating to observe, was
not only the transformation in my mother and myself,
but in everyone else at the Institute, as well.

There were about a hundred new guests every week
and we were meeting some amazing people from all
over the world. And they had every kind of physical
ailment that you could imagine - diabetes, arthritis,
skin disorders, thyroid conditions, obesity and tumors
and cancers of all varieties, just to name a few.

For most people, the first few days were challenging as they got used to the new regime and they were going through their initial purification.

But then, you could see the clarity in their eyes start to appear and the lightness in their step. Then after about the fifth day, after the juice fasting, everyone was a different version of them selves. They were more energetic and had more color in their cheeks. The dining room was much louder at meal times on these days, as people were much more alive and sociable.

Ann Wigmore shared this in her book – "In my years of working with this simple diet, I have observed that after following such a diet for a while, many people notice the disappearance of nagging problems they had lived with for months or years. Blocked sinuses open up, sleep is deeper and more restful, aches and pains are relieved, excess weight is quickly shed, the eyes become brighter, and facial stress disappears."

I was amazed at how this nurturing, dietary and cleansing program, not only was a powerful healer for cancer, but for every 'health opportunity' that there was – because once again – it is setting up the right healing environment for the body to self-heal from whatever was out of balance.

Friday Night Live

Then by Friday night everyone was so lively and ready for some action. So it is perfect that every week they hold a talent night, called 'Friday Night Live'. Anyone can sign up to get up on stage and entertain in whatever way they feel inclined to.

And there is usually some major talent that comes out and performs. It is always very surprising to see certain guests that you have been talking to all week, get up on stage and blow you away with an amazing talent. Like singing with a magnificent voice, or playing the piano in a gifted way. This talent show is one of my favorite things about Optimum and I look forward to it every time I go and I have even ventured up on stage myself, occasionally.

Shared Stories

"Strength does not come from physical capacity.
It comes from an indomitable will."
– Mahatma Ghandi

Another wonderful weekly ritual at OHI, is at the end of each week, everyone gathers together and anyone that wishes to, can share their story of healing.

At these meetings, I heard story, after story of how this program has helped people to heal from a diverse variety of conditions.

And the guests would express over and over again, how it has improved their quality of life, in so many ways. And in many instances, like my mother's, there were powerful stories of how the program has helped to save people's lives.

There was no denying the fact that this regime worked. And worked in a consistent and powerful way for people from all backgrounds, and from all over the world.

After the second week, I got up and told the story of my mother, as she was too shy to tell it herself. But I felt it was an important story to share, as it might inspire others in her shoes.

I couldn't help but cry, as I recounted what she had been through in such a short period of time. And when I looked around, everyone in the room had tears in their eyes, as well, even my mother, who was perhaps starting to realize all that she had been through.

I was able to express how much I loved and appreciated her and how strong and courageous I thought she had been throughout this whole experience.

After telling her story, my mother had so many people come up to her, wanting to hear more about her journey. And I think for the first time, it was really starting to sink in for her, what a traumatic and transformational experience it had all been for her. She had gone to the very edge of death and now was winning the battle against the most deadly of cancers.

Then she realized that it had been exactly three months since the doctor had told her that she was going to die. She had reached the three month marker and she was not only still alive, but she was feeling better than she had felt in years.

When we both realized this, we couldn't believe it! She was a walking, talking example of how you can actually heal from anything – even a disease that kills 97% of those that have it.

And she had done it completely naturally, without any western medical intervention whatsoever. Not even painkillers.

She was still fragile and had more healing to do, but she was no longer on her deathbed. In fact, her eyes were lit up with new life and her cheeks had a lovely pink glow. A far cry from only 12 weeks before, when her complexion was an eerie shade of green and her eyes expressed only excruciating pain and a fading life force.

I could not express enough how proud I was of her. It truly was her courage, focus and tenacity – that was the real reason she survived.

She showed me that you can be self-empowered about your health and there was no need to fear disease, even cancer, because we now knew the secrets of how to overcome it.

She really learned and transformed so much from both the Hippocrates Health Institute and the Optimum Health Institute. She was forever grateful to them both.

Raw People

I have to give mention, as well, to the staff members and teachers of the Optimum Health Institute. They all have such big hearts and are a big part of the wonderful warm atmosphere of the place.

One person in particular really stood out for my mother and I, though. He is a living example of the program and has been there since 1987. His name is Dan Strobhar and he has the biggest, purest heart of them all.

He does a little bit of everything at the Institute – from overseeing the organic garden and the wheat grass growing area, to teaching classes on yoga and wheat grass and talking to the guests on the phone.

He lives this program, every day, and is a radiant example of its effect. I have seen him there for over thirteen years and he hasn't aged a day.

He is such a wealth of knowledge and yet is the most humble person you would ever meet. I have learned so much from him every time I have gone, and I am grateful for his shining example of how to live a simple and raw life.

He says, "I really enjoy our guests and appreciate the determination and inspiration they bring to OHI. The transformation I see in people over a single week is amazing."

Thanks Dan!

Parting Ways

Once again it was time for my mother to go back home and continue this program on her own. This time, she was feeling much better, stronger, clearer, and with a new sense of empowerment over her health. She no longer felt like a victim to disease.

She now understood and knew what her body needed, to sustain health for the rest of her life. She no longer had a fear of cancer or death. She felt in control of her body and her life.

She was ready to step into her new life with all the new tools that she had been given.

It had been such a wonderful bonding time with my mother, who I thought I was losing, but instead I had this new found precious time with.

I was so grateful for the time spent with her and also for the transformations that I experienced in myself during the program.

What started out as a simple visit to the institute to help my mother, turned into a life transforming experience for myself. I felt like a new person and I was ready to go home and make some changes in my own life, to continue to feel good.

And so we had one last raw food meal together and wrapped up a meal to go and headed for the airport. It was hard for both of us to say good-bye to The Optimum Health Institute. We were both better versions of ourselves, by being there.

At the airport, I gave my mother the biggest hug and I didn't want to let go, but I had to let her move onto the next phase of her life. Tears of gratefulness flowed down my cheeks, as I watched her walk away and step into being - a vibrantly healthy and self-sufficient raw food, wheat grass woman of the world.

Way to go, Mom!

And this time, as I watched her walk away, I knew she was going to be just fine and I was going to be seeing her for many years to come.

Chapter Fourteen

A New Life

"Yesterday is gone. Tomorrow has not yet come.
We have only today. Let us begin."
– Mother Teresa

When Samantha went home this time, most things were already in place for her to start this new lifestyle on her own. She was prepared mentally and physically to fully incorporate this new regime in every way.

She had the kitchen appliances, the recipe books and she could have the wheat grass delivered right away.

And now she even had her Far Infrared "Hot House" Dome, which she immediately started using and has been using every day, twice a day, ever since. It's one thing she would never live without.

Samantha decided to adopt the regime of eating 80% live raw food and 20% cooked food. She felt that she could comfortably maintain this way of eating over a long period of time.

She wasn't perfect on the program all the time, but she was 100% vegetarian and ate very little processed food.

She made herself a special green drink every morning for breakfast (see the chapter 'Raw Recipes' – for her recipe). And she had fun being creative in making different varieties of salads, raw soups and other raw recipes.

When my mother ate cooked food, it was mostly freshly steamed brown rice, quinoa, lentils, chick peas and vegetables. And she did allow herself the occasional baked potato or sweet potato, as they were her favorites. But she had no more roast beef or other old favorites that made her feel worse, rather than better, afterwards.

She had wheat grass juice regularly and walked on her treadmill several times a week. She integrated completely into a new healthy routine that she was able to maintain comfortably everyday.

She was also able to go back to either Hippocrates or Optimum Institute about every six months.

Then before she knew it, it had been two years.

Two Years!

Samantha realized that she had made it to two years! She couldn't believe it, because when she first arrived at Hippocrates, all that time ago, and Brian Clement first talked about doing the program for two years, it seemed like an impossibility that she would be around that long.

But here she was! And when she thought back on how she felt when she first arrived there in 1999 and compared it to how she felt now, it was really true – she felt like she had remembered how to be healthy again and she had regained her strength and vitality.

The next time she was at Hippocrates she reminded Brian Clement of what he had told her. "If you follow this program to the letter, for two years, you will regain your health".

He was thrilled to see that she was still alive and doing so well. And was so impressed with her story that he not only put it in his monthly magazine, but printed it in his amazing book – "LifeForce". (It is available on Amazon.com)

Brian said that her story was so unusual, because it was rare that someone with Pancreatic Cancer had not had any Chemo, Radiation or surgery before coming to Hippocrates. And so she is the only guest that he has ever had up to that point, with this type of cancer, that had survived by purely natural means.

Brian asks my mother regularly, to talk on the phone with guests at Hippocrates that have Pancreatic Cancer. She is happy to do so and has inspired many people on their way to healing.

Even the American Cancer Society found her story intriguing and asked her for more information about it.

Samantha was once again reminded of how Dr. Brian Clement was instrumental in giving her another chance at life. And she will always be grateful and indebted to him for that.

Revisiting the Doctor

It was about at this two year mark that Samantha decided to go back to her doctor and see what was happening with her tumor.

Well, my mother said that she wished she took a picture of the expression on her doctor's face when she walked in the door. Her doctor had completely written her off for dead, two full years before and now, here she was, perfectly fine, up and walking around.

It took a moment for the doctor to come out of her stupor. She just kept looking at my mother's medical file and at the ultrasound picture from two years before, of the large 10cm tumor right on her pancreas.

She looked at my mother and at the ultrasound and scratched her head.

Samantha tried to explain what she had been doing, but because it didn't fit into the doctor's narrow view of how to treat cancer, the doctor didn't even hear a word my mother was saying.

Then the doctor mumbled something to herself, saying that there was no possible way that she could have survived this size of tumor, and at such an advanced stage.

And then my mother recalled the other thing that Brian Clement had said to her, on the first day that she arrived at Hippocrates – "And when you go back to your doctors, they won't believe that you're still alive and will probably say that you were misdiagnosed in the first place, even if they have the ultrasound of your tumor in their hands."

The doctor turned to my mother and said to her, "I'm so sorry, it appears that there must have been some mistake and we must have misdiagnosed you. I hope this did not cause you any inconvenience."

My mother laughed out loud when she heard this. She couldn't believe how predictable this was.

She assured the doctor that she did indeed have the tumor and she was there to see the size of it now. Still in shock, the doctor sent her off to do another ultrasound and an MRI, among other tests.

The ultrasound came back showing her tumor was still there, but it had shrunk to 4cm in diameter. The doctor saw that there was indeed still a tumor and she couldn't refute this evidence.

In fact the doctor said, that many people even with a 4cm size of a tumor on their pancreas usually don't last very long and are in great pain. So the fact that my mother was able to function normally with even this size of a mass, was amazing to her.

The doctor was baffled and didn't know what to tell my mother and so just told her to keep doing what she was doing, because it was working.

Thirteen Years & I'm Still Here!

"If you say you can, or you can't,
you are right either way ~ Henry Ford"

Well my mother did just that. She continued to do what she was doing and went back to Hippocrates and Optimum as often as she could.

She realized that if she continued to follow this lifestyle, that she would continue to live. It was not always easy for her, and it took focus and daily commitment to keep it up, but it was worth it.

Because she is still here, not only alive, but thriving, more than thirteen years after first being diagnosed!

Survival of any type of cancer is considered a success if you are alive even five years later. Well, my mother has defied the odds once again.

Who knows, she may even surprise us all, and reach her goal of "living to be a hundred".

Because my mother is still here, she has been able to watch my son, Jaydon , grow up to be a fine young man. She has been able to meet my niece, her new grand daughter, Skyla. And she even went on a cruise to Mexico and swam with the dolphins.

Back from the Edge of Death

Samantha experienced that cancer can be overcome, even the most deadly kind. Even when the top doctors in the country told her otherwise.

Coming back to life from the edge of death, shook her at her core and helped her to remove any fears about cancer or any illness, because now she knows what to do, to heal.

She learned that it makes no difference to the body, if we have a cut, a cold or cancer, the body does the same thing – it heals itself. Our body just needs the right environment to support it to do its job and it's possible to heal from anything.

My mother is a beacon of what is possible for anyone that has a serious illness. She is a walking, talking example that you can heal from anything, even when the odds are stacked against you and you are given only three months left to live.

She is living proof, without a doubt, that it is absolutely possible to survive - the death sentence of Pancreatic Cancer.

Summary

Here is a summary of all that my mother has learned in her thirteen year journey of healing.

The Most Important Thing - The body heals itself, no matter what the condition. It just needs to have the right environment to support itself to heal and it is possible for the body to heal from anything.

Creating the right healing conditions –

1) "Let Food be your Medicine and Medicine be your Food" – Eat as though your life depends on it, because it does – Eat a simple diet of 80% organic live raw foods and sprouts - for life force, enzymes, high nutrition and an alkaline environment

2) Cooked Food – 20% of diet - freshly prepared – steamed or baked – brown rice, quinoa, beans, lentils, vegetables

3) Breakfast – Fresh green vegetable juice or green drink – See Samantha's Morning Green Drink recipe – Recipe Chapter

4) Vegetable Juice Fasting – One day per week do a juice fast and it will keep your body clean and running smoothly

5) Wheat Grass Juice - "The Grass Factor" - Two ounces everyday - potent healing accelerator, highly nutritious, powerful detoxifier and creates an alkaline environment

6) Water – Stay hydrated – 100 trillion cells need lots of water to function at their best

7) Food Combining – Food digests better when combined properly

8) Foods to have Less of – All processed food, GMO foods, sugar, meat, dairy, pasta, bread, coffee, soda, alcohol

9) Alkaline (PH level) Environment – Cancer cells cannot survive in a highly alkaline environment – eat raw food, sprouts, wheat grass juice. No acidic food – meat, coffee, sugar, processed food

10) Oxygen Environment – Cancer cells cannot survive in a highly oxygenated environment and wheat grass juice has liquid oxygen that can easily be absorbed by the bloodstream

11) Stimulate the Immune System – Raw food, wheat grass juice, exercise, happy thoughts, laughing, doing something you love - all stimulate the immune system

12) Blood Sugar – Eat some protein every few hours to keep blood sugar levels balanced

13) Eating Habits – Eat slowly, chew your food well, only have happy thoughts when you are eating – you digest your thoughts

14) Exercise – "Stretch and Stroll" – Stretch and move your body around everyday for at least 30 minutes to keep the life energy flowing

15) Detoxify the Body regularly with massage, colonics, enemas and implants

16) Take Full Responsibility for your Health - Because you are responsible for it – nobody else is

17) Mental and Emotional Health – Let go and forgive old negative thoughts and emotions to create space for new joyful ones

18) Love, Laughter and Nurturing – Give and receive - hugs, smiles, jokes, kindness, caring, compliments - a happy heart creates happy cells in your body

19) Attitude of Healing – Positive attitude no matter what anyone else says and knowing that you can absolutely heal from anything

20) Attitude of Gratitude – Think of everything you are grateful for in your life and your heart will open and flow with love

21) Visualization – Use your imagination to picture yourself in excellent health

22) Daily Silence - Take a few minutes of inner quiet time to yourself everyday to reconnect with your spirit

23) Sleep – Get at least 8 hours per night

24) Bedtime – Lights out before 10:00pm - every hour that you get of sleep before 12:00am is worth 2 hours after 12:00am

25) Far Infrared Treatments – Detoxes the cells, increases blood circulation, stimulates the immune system and feels great! Samantha has been going under her "Hot House" everyday for 13 years

26) Energy Healing – Reiki, Healing Hands, Pranic Healing and other forms of energy healing, can work wonders in assisting the body to heal

27) And Most Importantly - Be yourself, everyone else is Taken.

I can never truly express how grateful I am that my mother is still around today.

She is a powerhouse of determination and courage and I love her and am deeply inspired by her, everyday.

I truly hope that my mother's story will inspire others, as well. And open up the possibility in people's hearts – that you can heal from anything. Even the death sentence, that is Pancreatic Cancer.

Chapter Fifteen

My Own Journey

*"Heaven is under our feet, as well as
over our heads." - Henry David Thoreau*

I was so transformed by my experience at the
Optimum Health Institute, that I have continued to go
back many times. I have now been there for over 14
weeks and I think of it as my second home.

Every time I go, I have deeper purifications and
realizations and I am able to integrate the program
more and more into my daily life.

I have also been to the Optimum Health Institute in
Austin, Texas. It is a smaller and more intimate
facility, set on several acres in a forest and has the
same program and classes as the San Diego one.

It is a lovely facility and setting, and I would recommend it for anyone desiring a quieter, more intimate experience.

Over time, most of my sisters have also gone to either the Hippocrates or Optimum Health Institutes and we have all integrated raw food more seriously into our lives. My mother's journey opened up all of our eyes to this new world.

Now when we get together, we have raw food potlucks and exchange raw food recipes and health tips. It has become a new way of life for all of us.

Raw Inspiration

Since being introduced to this wild and wonderful new world of Raw Food, I have come to find that there is a huge growing Raw Community out there. There is so much information now about it and these are a few Raw Food Leaders that have inspired me along the way.

David Wolfe

Known as the rock star of the raw food world. He has become a world renowned expert in everything to do with live raw and super foods. He has been one of the driving forces behind bringing the concept of raw food to the general public.

His discoveries of 'Super Foods' from around the world have now made it into most grocery stores.

Things like goji berries, raw cacao, maca powder, all come from his findings and promotions.

I have had the good fortune of seeing David speak live and he is a dynamo of energy and clarity. David empowers and inspires people to take charge of their own health because, after all, as he likes to say, "Health is Wealth!"

Books – The Sunfood Diet Success System; Naked Chocolate; Eating for Beauty; Superherbs; Superfoods

Website - http://www.davidwolfe.com

Victoria Boutenko

She has written one of my favorite raw books – 'Raw Family' – about the story of her family when they first moved to the USA from Russia and became very ill from eating the wrong foods. Then Victoria discovered raw food and her family completely recovered from diabetes, obesity, depression and other ailments. It is a great book to give someone to introduce them to the idea and world of raw food.

Books – Raw Family; Green Smoothie Revolution; 12 Steps to Raw Foods; Green for Life; Raw and Beyond

Website - http://www.rawfamily.com

Dr. Gabriel Cousens

Dr. Gabriel Cousens is considered one of the leading live-food medical doctors and spiritual nutrition experts in the world, and, is recognized as "the fasting guru and detoxification expert" by the New York Times. He is also a psychiatrist, family therapist, Ayurvedic practitioner, homeopath and acupuncturist.

I have had the good fortune of being a guest at Dr. Cousen's - Tree of Life Rejuvenation Center - in Patagonia, Arizona. It is a wonderful retreat center that combines ancient Ayurvedic treatments with a Raw Food diet. The food at the center is gourmet raw food at its best and is exceptionally delicious.

Dr. Cousens also specializes in green juice fasting and the more spiritual aspects of a raw lifestyle. He is an inspirational speaker and a wealth of knowledge on all things raw and is one of the great leaders in this field.

Books – Spiritual Nutrition; Conscious Eating; Creating Peace By Being Peace; Depression-Free for Life; Rainbow Green Live Food Cuisine; There is a Cure for Diabetes

Center – Tree of Life Rejuvenation Center – Patagonia, AZ

Website - http://www.treeoflife.nu

Chapter Sixteen

Raw Recipes

Samantha's Morning Green Drink

Put in blender, blend until smooth and enjoy!

1 cup – Filtered Water
2-6 - Ice Cubes
1 handful - Fresh Organic Raw Baby Spinach
1 Organic Banana
¼ tspn – Organic Maca Powder,
1 small handful – Organic Goji Berries,
1-2 tbspn – Organic Raw Cacao Powder,
2 tbspn – Organic Raw Protein Powder (non-soy),

Optimum Health Institute

Here are some great 100% raw recipes from the
Optimum Health Institute – Thank-you OHI!
Enjoy!

Basic Green Juice
Yields about 2 quarts

1 bunch	Celery
2 each	Cucumbers
1 each	Zucchini
¼ head	Cabbage
½ bunch	Swiss Chard
½ bunch	Kale
1 cup fresh chopped	Fennel
1 small piece of fresh	Ginger
Any type of sprouts	
Any leafy green vegetables	

Seasoning to taste
Dulce and Powered Kelp

Add to Basic Juice
1 small Beets
¼ head red cabbage
2 Carrots

Tomato Bisque Soup
Yields 2 -3 servings

6 -7 pureed	Tomatoes
¼ cup	Tomato powder
2 pureed	Avocados
1 finely minced	Garlic cloves
1 tablespoon finely chopped	Basil
2 tablespoons granulated	Kelp
2 tablespoons powdered	Celery

Place all ingredients in food processor or blend.
Combine until smooth.

Cucumber Soup
Yields 7 or 8 – 8 oz servings

10 peeled	Cucumbers
3 each pitted	Avocados
1 cups ground	Pine nuts
½ teaspoon	Mexican seasoning

Place cucumbers and scooped out avocados in
the food processor. Combine until smooth.
Add ground pine nuts blending until smooth.
Add Mexican seasoning.

Guacamole/ Avocado Dressing

Yields about 2 cups

2 each mashed	Avocado
1 chopped	Tomato
½ chopped	Yellow onions
2 each chopped	Green onions
1 small bunch chopped	Cilantro
1 teaspoon	Mexican seasoning
1 teaspoon	Kelp
1 teaspoon	Cumin

Mix all ingredients in large bowl. Place several pits
of the avocado in bowl to keep from turning brown.
Remove pit before serving.

For Avocado Dressing -

Use same ingredients and put into blender until
Consistency is that of dressing. Do the same with the
pits of the avocados.

Tomato Basil Salad Dressing
Yields about 1 quart

10 blended	Tomatoes
1 teaspoon powdered	Garlic
¼ cup finely chopped	Basil
1 ounces	Apple cider vinegar
½ cup	Tomato powder

Combined all ingredients in food processor or blender
until smooth

Coleslaw
Yields about 6 servings

1 head slaw or chopped	Cabbage
2 diced	Tomatoes
1 chopped	Avocado
3 each diced	Green onions

1 tablespoon chopped	Parsley

Dressing:

1 cup finely ground	Pines Nut
¼ cup	Water
¼ inch finely chopped	Ginger
½ cup finely chopped	Celery
1 tablespoon powdered	Kelp
1 teaspoon dried	Dill weed
1/8 teaspoon	Cayenne

Combine first 5 ingredients in large bowl and set aside

Dressing:

Place pine nuts in food processor adding water a little at a time.

Add ginger and celery until smooth.

Add kelp, dill weed, and cayenne until mixed.

Pour dressing over large bowl set aside.

Flax Seed Crackers

Yields 3 – 4 dehydration trays

¼ cup chopped	Onions
1 diced	Tomato
1 small clove	Garlic
1 cup soaked	Flax seeds
½ teaspoon	Cumin or chili powder

Optional Ingredient   finely chopped Cilantro

Put garlic and onions in food processor until smooth. Add tomato until blended.
Put mixture into large bowl, add flax seeds and seasoning

Place measured tablespoon of mixture 3 to 4 across and 3 to 4 down on the tray. Tap tray lightly until mixture spread into circles.

Dehydrate under 105 degrees until crispy (2- 2 ½ days)

Nori rolls – (Raw Sushi)
Yields 20 to 24 pieces

5 sheets	Nori
1 cup	Seed cheese
½ cup shredded	Carrots
½ cup diced	Celery
1 cup	Alfalfa Sprouts
1 cup sprouted	Sunflower sprouts
1 julienne sliced	Red pepper
1 cup finely chopped	Cucumber

Divide seed cheese into 5 portions
Spread seed cheese on nori than layer with carrots, celery, alfalfa sprouts, buckwheat spouts, red peppers, cucumber.
Roll like a California Roll
Cut into 4 or 6 pieces

Mock Spaghetti & Meatballs

Spaghetti Sauce

3 pureed	Tomatoes
1 finely ground	Carrot
1 finely chopped	Fresh basil
1 pureed	Red Pepper
1 tablespoon	Italian Seasoning
½ tspn granulated	Kelp

Add tomato powder to thicken.

Spaghetti Noodles

2 medium	Zucchini

Use a Universal Equipment Machine
Spiral Attachment

Mock Meatballs
Yields approximately 12 -15 meatballs

1 finely chopped	Zucchini
1 finely chopped	Carrot
½ diced	Red Peppers
½ chopped	Onion
2 sprigs chopped	Parsley
1 clove finely chopped	Garlic
½ teaspoon dried	Oregano

1 tablespoon dry or fresh	Basil
1/4 teaspoon dried	Cloves
1/2 teaspoon	Marjoram
1/4 teaspoon dry or fresh	Rosemary (ground)
1 tablespoon	Celery powder
1 tablespoon	Tomato powder
1 teaspoon powdered	Kelp
1/2 teaspoon	Cumin
½ teaspoon	Chili powder
½ cup finely ground	Pumpkin seeds

Mix all ingredients and form into a ball

Chapter Seventeen

More Information

I have included some more information on many aspects that we have covered in this book, for those that may be interested.

Food Combining Guide

The basic concept of food combining is – that there are different digestive fluids or gastric acids that are required to digest different foods. For example – there is a different fluid needed to digest protein, than there is to digest fruit. So if you eat protein with fruit at the same time, then neither of these foods gets digested properly.

So it is best to eat certain foods separately from other foods, like - fruit, melons, wheat grass juice. Eat these foods alone and allow some time for them to digest before eating other foods.

Then it is okay to combine other foods together -
- Green vegetables and sprouts can basically be
combined with almost all foods, except fruit.
- Dense proteins – avocados, nuts, seeds and beans,
can be combined with only green vegetables and
sprouts
- Starchy vegetables and grains, like potatoes and
brown rice, cannot be combined with proteins, but
can be combined with green vegetables.

There are a lot more details about this and for a
complete chart go to my website -
http://www.sistergoddesssanctuary.com

The Hot House

One thing that my mother has continued to do, for
thirteen years, is to go under her beloved "Hot
House" every single day. She also discovered the
"Chi Machine" about eight years ago, which helps
increase circulation and the flow of oxygen in the
body, and she does both machines together, morning
and night. (For more information on the "Hot House"
and "Chi Machine" – visit her website -
http://www.htesoqi.com/samanthayoung

The Benefits of Wheat Grass Juice
(From the Hippocrates Health Institute)

I thought I would include more information about wheat grass juice. This is a detailed list of things that wheat grass has been shown to have an effect on.

This is not a scientific list, but it comes from the Hippocrates Health Institute, where they have been observing the effects of wheat grass for over 50 years.

Wheat Grass Juice –

Increases red blood-cell count and lowers blood pressure. It cleanses the blood, organs and gastrointestinal tract of debris. Wheatgrass also stimulates metabolism and the body's enzyme systems by enriching the blood. It also aids in reducing blood pressure by dilating the blood pathways throughout the body.

Stimulates the thyroid gland, correcting obesity, indigestion, and a host of other complaints.

Restores alkalinity to the blood. The juice's abundance of alkaline minerals helps reduce over-acidity in the blood. It can be used to relieve many internal pains, and has been used successfully to treat peptic ulcers, ulcerative colitis, constipation, diarrhea, and other complaints of the gastrointestinal tract.

Is a powerful detoxifier, and liver and blood protector. The enzymes and amino acids found in wheatgrass can protect us from carcinogens like no other food or medicine. It strengthens our cells, detoxifies the liver and bloodstream, and chemically neutralizes environmental pollutants.

Fights tumors and neutralizes toxins. Recent studies show that wheatgrass juice has a powerful ability to fight tumors without the usual toxicity of drugs that also inhibit cell-destroying agents. The many active compounds found in grass juice cleanse the blood and neutralize and digest toxins in our cells.

Contains beneficial enzymes. Whether you have a cut finger you want to heal or you desire to lose five pounds…enzymes must do the actual work. The life and abilities of the enzymes found naturally in our bodies can be extended if we help them from the outside by adding exogenous enzymes, like the ones found in wheatgrass juice. Don't cook it. We can only get the benefits of the many enzymes found in grass by eating it uncooked. Cooking destroys 100 percent of the enzymes in food.

Has remarkable similarity to our own blood. The second important nutritional aspect of chlorophyll is its remarkable similarity to hemoglobin, when the "blood" of plants is absorbed in humans it is transformed into human blood, which transports nutrients to every cell of the body.

When used as a rectal implant, reverses damage from inside the lower bowel. An implant is a small amount of juice held in the lower bowel for about 20 minutes. In the case of illness, wheatgrass implants stimulate a rapid cleansing of the lower bowel and draw out accumulations of debris.

Externally applied to the skin can help eliminate itching almost immediately.

Will soothe sunburned skin and act as a disinfectant. Rubbed into the scalp before a shampoo, it will help mend damaged hair and alleviate itchy, scaly, scalp conditions.

Is soothing and healing for cuts, burns, scrapes, rashes, poison ivy, athlete's foot, insect bites, boils, sores, open ulcers, tumors, and so on. Use as a poultice and replace every two to four hours.

Works as a sleep aide. Merely place a tray of living wheatgrass near the head of your bed. It will enhance the oxygen in the air and generate healthful negative ions to help you sleep more soundly.

Enhances your bath. Add some to your bath water and settle in for a nice, long soak.

Sweetens the breath and firms up and tightens gums. Just gargle with the juice.

Neutralizes toxic substances like cadmium, nicotine, strontium, mercury, and polyvinyl chloride.

Offers the benefits of a liquid oxygen transfusion since the juice contains liquid oxygen. Oxygen is vital to many body processes: it stimulates digestion (the oxidation of food), promotes clearer thinking (the brain utilizes 25% of the body's oxygen supply), and protects the blood against anaerobic bacteria. Cancer cells cannot exist in the presence of oxygen.

Turns gray hair to its natural color again and greatly increases energy levels when consumed daily.

Is a beauty treatment that slows down the aging process when the juice is consumed. Wheatgrass will cleanse your blood and help rejuvenate aging cells, slowing the aging process way down, making you feel more alive right away. It will help tighten loose and sagging skin.

Lessens the effects of radiation. One enzyme found in wheatgrass, SOD, lessens the effects of radiation and acts as an anti-inflammatory compound that may prevent cellular damage following heart attacks or exposure to irritants.

Restores fertility and promotes youthfulness.

Can double your red blood cell count just by soaking in it. Renowned nutritionist Dr. Bernard Jensen found that no other blood builders are superior to green juices and wheatgrass.

In his book Health Magic Through Chlorophyll from Living Plant Life he mentions several cases where he was able to double the red blood cell count in a matter of days merely by having patients soak in a chlorophyll-water bath. Blood building results occur even more rapidly when patients drink green juices and wheatgrass regularly.

Reference and Recommended Books

'Why Suffer - How I Overcame Illness and Pain Naturally' – Ann Wigmore
http://www.amazon.com/Why-Suffer-Overcame-Illness-Naturally/dp/0895292866

- Ann Wigmore's personal story of how she discovered the healing power of wheat grass juice and used it to help herself and countless others to heal themselves naturally.

'Man's Search for Meaning' - Viktor Frankl
http://www.amazon.com/Mans-Search-Meaning-Viktor-Frankl/dp/080701429X

- Psychiatrist Viktor Frankl's memoir has riveted generations of readers with its descriptions of life in Nazi death camps and its lessons for spiritual survival.

'You Can Heal Your Life' – Louise Hay
http://www.louisehay.com

- Louise Hay discovered that there were common underlying mental/emotional components to each type of physical ailment and she documented these correlations. This book is a wonderful compilation of her findings.

'The China Study' - Dr. T. Colin Campbell and Thomas M. Campbell II
http://www.thechinastudy.com

- In The China Study, Dr. T. Colin Campbell details the connection between nutrition and heart disease, diabetes, and cancer. The New York Times has recognized the study as the "Grand Prix of epidemiology" and the "most comprehensive large study ever undertaken of the relationship between diet and the risk of developing disease."

Inspirational Raw Food Leaders/Books

David Wolfe –

Books – The Sunfood Diet Success System; Naked Chocolate; Eating for Beauty; Superherbs: Super Foods

Website - http://www.davidwolfe.com

Victoria Boutenko

Books – Raw Family; Green Smoothie Revolution;
12 Steps to Raw Foods; Green for Life; Raw and
Beyond

Website - http://www.rawfamily.com

Dr. Gabriel Cousens

Books – Spiritual Nutrition; Conscious Eating;
Creating Peace By Being Peace; Depression-Free for
Life; Rainbow Green Live Food Cuisine; There is a
Cure for Diabetes

Center – Tree of Life Rejuvenation Center

Website - http://www.treeoflife.nu

Inspirational Videos

These are a few videos that have opened my eyes and
have changed the way I look at a lot of things.

'Forks Over Knives' –
Creator and Executive Producer - Brian Wendel
http://www.forksoverknives.com

'Fat Sick and Nearly Dead' –
Producer/Director – Joe Cross
http://www.fatsickandnearlydead.com

'Food Inc' –
Producer/Director - Robert Kenner
http://www.takepart.com/foodinc

Reference Websites

The Hippocrates Health Institute –
http://www.hippocratesinst.org

The Optimum Health Institute –
http://www.optimumhealth.org

The Real Truth About Health -
http://therealtruthabouthealth.com.

David Wolfe
http://www.davidwolfe.com

Raw Family
http://www.rawfamily.com

Hypnosis Motivation Institute
https://www.hypnosis.edu

Cancer Fighting Strategies –
http://cancerfightingstrategies.com/oxygen-and-cancer.html

Well + Good, NYC
http://www.wellandgoodnyc.com

HuffPost Healthy Living
http://www.huffingtonpost.com

EFT
http://eft.mercola.com/
http://www.rogercallahan.com/index2.php

Wikipedia
http://www.wikipedia.org

Ann Wigmore
http://www.whale.to/a/wigmore_q.html

GoodReads
www.goodreads.com

Sister Goddess Sanctuary
http://www.sistergoddesssanctuary.net

Samantha Young's Website -
http://www.htesoqi.com/samanthayoung

I

Information on the Health Institutes

Hippocrates Health Institute

Website - http://www.hippocratesinst.org

Call to make a reservation - 1-800-842-2125

Address –

1465 Skees Rd.
West Palm Beach
Florida 33411

Dr. Brian Clement's Website -
http://therealtruthabouthealth.com.

Optimum Health Institute

Website - http://www.optimumhealth.org

Call to make a reservation - 1-800-993-4325

San Diego, California address -

6970 Central Avenue
Lemon Grove, CA 91945

Austin, Texas address –

265 Cedar Lane
Cedar Creek, TX 78612

Our Websites

Samantha Young's Website -
http://www.htesoqi.com/samanthayoung

Traysiah Spring's Website –
http://www.sistergoddesssanctuary.com

Wishing you a thriving, joyful life!

22921547R00083

Made in the USA
Lexington, KY
19 May 2013